The Sasquatch, The Yowie, and the Spiral Butte Killers
and other writings
by Bob Reddick

The Sasquatch, The Yowie, and the Spiral Butte Killers and other writings by Bob Reddick

Published by Bob Reddick, Kenmore, Washington, USA

Copyright © 2021 by Bob Reddick. All Rights Reserved.

Cover art by Rob Dunlavey

ISBN: 9798614404321

Send email regarding this book to rogainer@xoc.net.

Original publication dates:

Olympic Simultaneous. ©1976. *Chess Life & Review* July 1976 in the Reader's Showcase.
Nettles in the Knees. ©1987. *Bearing 315*. Article I published in *Orienteering North America* January 1988.
Dragnet Rogaine '88. ©1988. *Orienteering North America* July 1988.
The (Pre-Swedish) History of Orienteering. ©1988. *Orienteering North America* November 1988.
The Pontius Arrowhead. ©1989. *Orienteering North America* June 1989.
Orienteers Need Water–Seriously. ©1989. *Orienteering North America* July 1989.
Three Navigation Books. ©1989. *Orienteering North America* November 1989.
Are You Ready for White? ©1990. *Orienteering North America* January 1990.
Orienteering Word Puzzle. ©1990. *Orienteering North America* January 1990, with solution in the August 1990 issue.
O-Atlas Washington State and Puget Sound. ©1990. *Orienteering North America* July 1990.
A Change in Competitive Style. ©1992. *Bearing 315* November/December 1992.
Rogaine Planning Plus an Invitation. ©1993. *Orienteering North America* March/April 1993.
Reddick's Rogaine Ruminations. ©1993. *Orienteering North America* June 1993.
Table Mountain Rogaine. ©1993. *Bearing 315* September 1993.
Rogaining Pet Theories. ©1993. Privately circulated letter dated September 30, 1993.
Interview. ©1994. *IRB Bulletin #2*.
The Spiral Butte Mishap. ©1994-1995. *Orienteering North America* November 1994 though May 1995 issues.
Science Olympiad. ©1995 by Larry Berman and Bob Reddick. *Orienteering North America* February 1995.
Surviving Your First Rogaine. ©1995. *Bearing 315* May 1995.
Shocking News: True Origin of Rogaining Revealed! ©1995. *Orienteering North America* July 1995.
Rogainer Almost Does Last Relocation. ©1996. *Bearing 315* May 1996.
Who Owns the Aardvark? ©1996. *Orienteering North America* August 1996.
Arizona Rogaine. ©1997. *Orienteering North America* April 1997.
Rogaine Food. ©1997. *Bearing 315* September/October 1997.
World Master Games: How I Lost My Gold Medal. ©1998. *Orienteering North America* October 1998.
1999 Nor-Am Rogaine Champs Critique & Etc. ©1999. *Orienteering North America* July 1999.
Elkhorn Rogaine = Challenging Terrain. ©2000. *Orienteering North America* November 2000.
Vergillo, Groff Clean the Map at First US Metrogaine, Held in Bremerton, WA ©2003. *Orienteering North America* July/August 2003.
The Australian Pursuit. ©2003. *Orienteering North America* April through October 2003 issues.
Black Hills WRC Search and Rescue For Real. ©2014. *Orienteering North America* September/October 2014.

Images:

Southern Cassowary by Snowmanradio CC BY-SA 2.0 https://creativecommons.org/licenses/by-sa/2.0/
Solar Glory by Brocken Inaglory CC-BY-SA 3.0 https://creativecommons.org/licenses/by-sa/3.0/
Comet Hale-Bopp by Philipp Salzgeber CC-BY-SA-2.0-AT https://creativecommons.org/licenses/by-sa/2.0/at/deed.en

The Kiwi.

*For Pat, who shared these many adventures
with me...loved the travel, new friends, and events,
but not the courses.*

A society grows great when old men plant trees
in whose shade they know they shall never sit

Table of Contents

INTRODUCTION ... 1
THE SPIRAL BUTTE MISHAP – A Rogaining Misadventure ... 2
THE AUSTRALIAN PURSUIT – A Rogaining Misadventure ... 26
ORIENTEERING CONTROL SIGNAGE ... 50
OLYMPIC SIMULTANEOUS ... 51
NETTLES IN THE KNEES I ... 52
NETTLES IN THE KNEES II – Route Selection ... 55
NETTLES IN THE KNEES III ... 58
NETTLES IN THE KNEES IV ... 60
NETTLES IN THE KNEES V – Night Orienteering ... 63
DRAGNET ROGAINE '88 ... 65
THE (PRE-SWEDISH) HISTORY OF ORIENTEERING ... 68
THE PONTIUS ARROWHEAD ... 69
ORIENTEERS NEED WATER–SERIOUSLY – A Competitor's, Meet Director's, and Course-Setter's Guide ... 70
BOOK REVIEWS – Three Navigation Books ... 73
ARE YOU READY FOR WHITE? – Ideas for the Competitor and the Designer ... 75
ORIENTEERING WORD PUZZLE ... 80
O-ATLAS – Washington State and Puget Sound ... 81
A CANOE O' ... 83
A CHANGE IN COMPETITIVE STYLE ... 84
ROGAINE PLANNING – Plus an Invitation ... 86
REDDICK'S ROGAINE RUMINATIONS ... 89
TABLE MOUNTAIN ROGAINE ... 92
ROGAINING PET THEORIES ... 95
INTERVIEW ... 96
YOUNGSTERS IN THE BACK YARD ... 98
SCIENCE OLYMPIAD – Where You Can Help Youngsters Get Involved in Navigation Sports ... 99
SURVIVING YOUR FIRST ROGAINE – How to Do It Right the First Time ... 101
SHOCKING NEWS: True Origins of Rogaining Revealed! ... 103
ROGAINER ALMOST DOES LAST RELOCATION ... 105

WHO OWNS THE AARDVARK? Rogaining Puzzle for Those Temporally Unchallenged................106
ARIZONA ROGAINE – North American Championships: March 1-2......................107
ROGAINE FOOD 113
WORLD MASTERS GAMES – How I Lost My Gold Medal..................................115
1999 NOR-AM ROGAINE – Critique & Etc..117
ELKHORN ROGAINE = CHALLENGING TERRAIN..118
VERGILLO, GROFF CLEAN THE MAP AT FIRST US METROGAINE, Held in Bremerton, WA.............122
NEIL AND ROD PHILLIPS AWARDED MEDAL OF THE ORDER OF AUSTRALIA.......................126
FIGMENT?..127
ROGAINING EXCUSE T-SHIRT..128
ORDER OF THE GEODUCK 129
BLACK HILLS WRC SEARCH AND RESCUE—FOR REAL...130

INTRODUCTION

In early 1994 while organizing the Spiral Butte Rogaine, I drafted a one-page ad to promote the event in Orienteering/North America magazine. Describing the terrain, I tried to bring a possible Sasquatch sighting in to attract potential competitors but found just one page too limiting. So, I called the editor, Sara Mae Berman, to chat about the ad. She said she loved serials, having printed Wilf Holloway's mystery back in 1987 as a serial. With her go-ahead, I began a six-part serial interactive mystery story, which was followed nine years later by its sequel.

I used fictitious names for all characters but borrowed and mixed up first and last names of active rogainers from several countries.

At 2 AM one night I awoke during the writing of an early chapter of Spiral Butte Mishap. My brain had brought up a memory of a short film I'd seen on November 26th, 1952 (my birthday) on Alistair Cooke's Omnibus TV show. The Seattle Public Library and the UW library reference librarians helped me find that award-winning film, "The Stranger Left No Card" (still seeable on YouTube). That was where my plot device came from. I also asked readers to add to my interactive story after each issue, and several did.

Then there was the continual research to find the many sayings, photos, the kangaroo tail soup recipe, etc. Most revealing for this new fiction writer was having to read three books and call a search-and-rescue dog training school to get accurate info for Boomer's short entry. Artists Rob Dunlavey and Rich Vail added clever renderings of the two legendary title characters, and Rob did most of the other art, including the cover.

The other writings over 33 years of competing and organizing orienteering, rogaining, and metrogaine events, some puzzles, and even a chess game, were lots of fun, including the subtle humor in casting doubt on the real history of these great sports. You will see that two originators were properly recognized by their country with the prestigious Order of Australia.

I have hopes that my small contributions of the 10-lb. pack rule, the collective noun "quest" for a bunch of navigators, the Geoduck Awards for organizers, and the push for EYE LEVEL control bag hanging will prevail.

I have many memories, mostly good, of fine courses, great people, enduring partners, two heart attacks, three first places, and only one DNF, one mis-mapped control, and no blood, broken bones, or serious blisters.

Partners who have left us for a better venue include "Mac" MacDonald, Knut Olson, Al Smith, Bruce McAlister, and Ken Lew. Thanks to all of you still here enjoying these great sports, and for your contributions to these articles.

This book was intended to be given as an added award to each of the ninety-plus team members winning in their classes at the World Rogaining Championships in August 2020 at Lake Tahoe, CA. This event, capping the 10-event Cal-O-Fest, was postponed to August 2021 by the world-wide novel coronavirus Covid-19 pandemic.

Acknowledgements

Thanks are given to Rob Dunlavey who did much of the original art that was included with the articles, as well as a new drawing for the cover of the book. Rich Vail did the drawings in The Australian Pursuit.

THE SPIRAL BUTTE MISHAP –
A Rogaining Misadventure

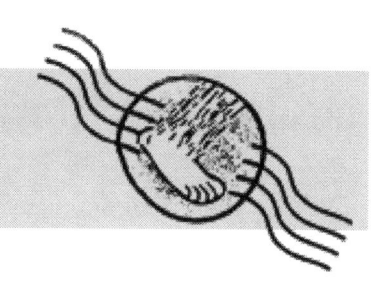

PART I – The Fall

The story you're about to read is not true. The names have been changed and scrambled to protect the innocent, who sometimes rogaine. The narrative times are from the detective's notes. Direct quotations are recorded where appropriate.

DUM DE DUM DUM, DUM DE DUM DUM, DUMMMM. *(The reader must intone this theme music aloud, for proper effect—or the story may not work! For those of you born after the 1950s, ask your older relatives about an early TV police show called DRAGNET.)*

It was a hot August afternoon. My partner Carl Newson and I were working the weekend watch out of the West Yakima Precinct. The boss is Captain Bruce Lawhead. My name's NotFriday. I carry a badge, number 714. We got a call from Ardis Newell at the Naches Ranger Station. She told us that there'd been an accident on Spiral Butte near White Pass, and a man was dead. Foul play was a suspected. My job: find the killer, if there is one.

4:10 PM. In Yakima, Carl and I swapped our sedan for the air-conditioned Land Cruiser from the drug patrol unit and headed out on Highway 12 to White Pass. It took us one hour of hard driving to get to the Dog Lake Campground. Some sort of sports event called a "rogaine" was going on. We introduced ourselves to the officials. They told us that one team member from Rogaine Team #13, a Mr. Knut Phillips, had apparently fallen near the top of Spiral Butte Sunday morning, and had been found dead. They thought we should be called to investigate, even though it appeared to be a tragic accident.

5:20 PM. We talked to the meet director, a Mr. Rick Landchild, at their event center tent (called a Hash House). He explained that this event involved long-distance navigation and endurance with a map and compass. In this case, the event covered about 100 square kilometers, or some 40 square miles of mountainous terrain, an area of rugged alpine meadow and evergreen forest,

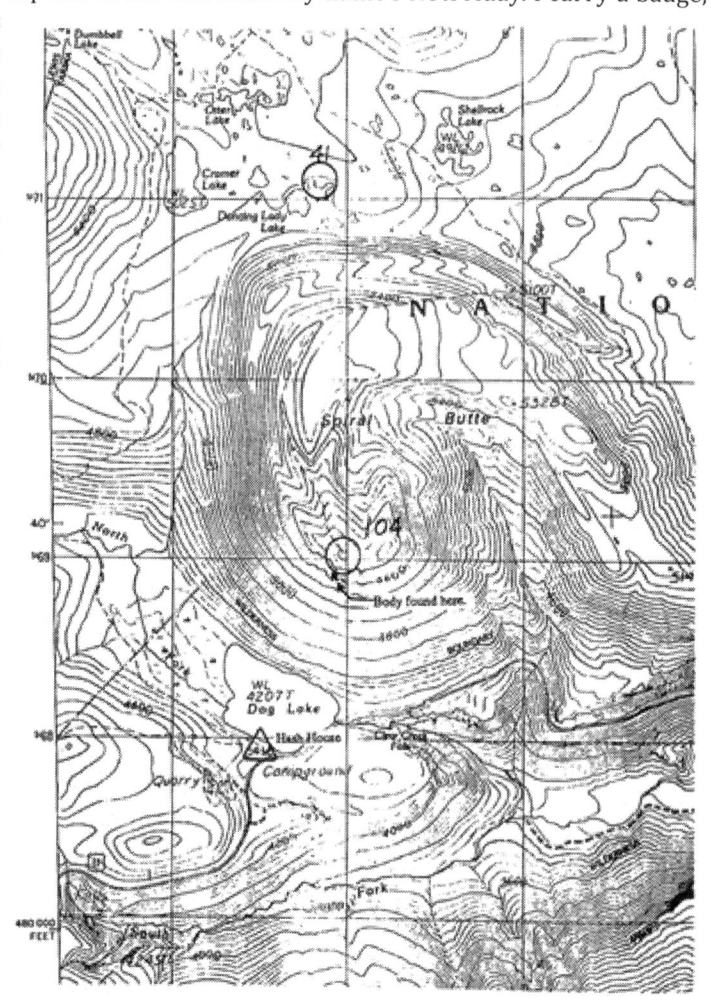

Published in *Orienteering North America* November 1994 through May 1995 issues.

called the William O. Douglas Wilderness. This area is part of the Snoqualmie National Forest, also in the Gifford Pinchot National Forest, and to complicate matters further, both are in Lewis County and Yakima County, Washington State. By arrangement, our police jurisdiction included investigation of deaths in these Federal lands.

Sixty teams had taken part in this rogaine. Each team had two to five members—some 131 people in all. Landchild called this assembly of rogainers a "quest," and started to go on about the usual mass start, etc., but I cut him short and asked about the accident. He said that Mr. Phillips, the deceased, had started out at noon on Saturday with his partner, Wyatt Fulton, and had nearly completed the event when the fatality occurred. Landchild told us that each team chooses its own route and decides which controls, or locations they will try to find within the 24 hours. He showed us the standard USGS 1:24,000 scale map that each person was issued. The 55 control locations were circled on it, plus the triangle for the start (and finish) at the Hash House location here at Dog Lake Campground.

At each control they punch a control card with a special kind of paper punch (each with its own pattern) to prove they've been there. They also sign in on an "Intention Sheet" hanging there. This is a log showing time of arrival, number of the team, signatures of all members, and the control number of the

CONTROL NUMBER: 41			INTENTION SHEET	DANCING LADY LAKE
Approved for hanging here by USFS-SNF.			Event in progress - DO NOT REMOVE	
Time	Team #	Next Control	Names	Signatures
(Previous day's and late night entries -- irrelevant)				
08:01	22	104	Kim Stark/Kent Ellsworth	(sigs. all checked OK)
08:25	13	104	Knut Phillips/Wyatt Fulton	
08:26	3	104	Peter Waugh/Fred Hudson	
08:28	1	104	Les Petty/Scott MacDonald	
09:30	54	HH	Urban Family (4)	
(no other entries)				

CONTROL NUMBER: 104			INTENTION SHEET	SPIRAL BUTTE
Approved for hanging here by USFS-SNF.			Event in progress - DO NOT REMOVE	
Time	Team #	Next Control	Names	Signatures
(Previous day's entries -- irrelevant)				
10:01	3	HH	Peter Waugh/Fred Hudson	(signatures checked against
10:03	22	HH	Kim Stark/Kent Ellsworth	registration waivers; all OK;
10:06	13	HH	Knut Phillips/Wyatt Fulton	not reproduced here)
10:10	1	HH	Les Petty/Scott MacDonald	
(blank)				

Here are the finish times and results compiled at the HH:

Tm #	Time in	Total Pts	Penalty pts.	Net Points	Position in Class
(Other returning teams -- irrelevant)					
13	11:56	DNF - Phillips not in		(no punch card)	?
3	12:02	2550	-2*10=20	2530	First Place overall & Masters
1	12:08	1840 PTS	- 8*10=80	1760 PTS	Third Place - Masters Class
22	12:50	1640 PTS	- 50*10=500	1140 PTS	Fourth Place - Mixed Class

next control they "intend" to visit. Landchild explained that the intention sheets are a safety factor in case a team is reported overdue or lost, to help establish just where they've been and when. He explained that while waiting for us to arrive, he'd recovered and reviewed the Spiral Butte Intention Sheet, and asked all teams who'd been there today to not leave the area. We asked if we could review these sheets. Landchild said that besides the Spiral Butte log, the one from Dancing Lady Lake had been recovered, showing Team 13's entries. A few of the rest were available if needed, having been recovered by teams volunteering for a "One Control Pickup". Landchild also warned us that they might not get all the Intention Sheets back, since some had been reported torn down and already missing. Deer and some other big-footed creatures seem to be attracted to them.

Landchild said that he had a bad feeling about this accident. Fulton came in just before the 12 noon deadline time, and asked if his partner, Phillips, had checked in yet, Landchild told him no, and asked when he had seen him last.

"You see, team members are never supposed to separate out of earshot," Landchild said. "It is quite irregular for one person to come in alone. Wyatt told me that they left the last control at the top of Spiral Butte together, but had become separated in descending the very steep volcanic cone's hillside. When he reached the bottom at the far shore of Dog Lake, he had called to his partner, but got no answer. Since it was almost noon, and serious penalty points are assessed for returning late, he figured his partner was running in, expecting him to be doing the same." So Fulton ran in. "We recorded him in at 11:56 AM. That team would have been the overall winner if this hadn't happened."

I asked, "Any big prizes involved?" Landchild replied, "Ha! Not in rogaining. We gave out the ribbons about 12:30, except for the mixed class, which was final at 12:50. Oh, but we do have one big sponsor, K*Swiss. They were considering an endorsement contract and world promotional tour for the winning team. So, I guess you might say there were big dollars at stake here."

Carl interjected, "I'd take a world tour any day to my Yakima job!"

I asked Dave Carroll about the search for Mr. Phillips. Carroll, the chief of the local search and rescue team, reported that he had organized three teams at about 1 PM to begin a search. All the other competing rogaine teams had returned, and several rogainers volunteered to join the teams. Dr. Scott MacDonald was the first to volunteer. For an orienteer and rogainer as experienced and fit as Phillips, the longest time it should have taken him to reach the Hash House, even allowing for mistakes, was about 2 hours and 15 minutes. Three search teams set off—one going the long way to the far side of Spiral Butte, then to the top via the trail. The other two went opposite ways around Dog Lake to search the shoreline and the routes that lead up the volcanic slopes. The lifeless body was found at about 3:30 PM by MacDonald and Deputy Sheriff Linda Jones near the top of the mountain, at the foot of a nearly sheer 50-foot rocky bluff. Phillips's skull was badly fractured; there were no other obvious injuries. Carroll called for an ambulance via radio, and had the Naches Ranger Station call Yakima Police Headquarters. Miss Kim Stark identified the body. The ambulance took Phillips'

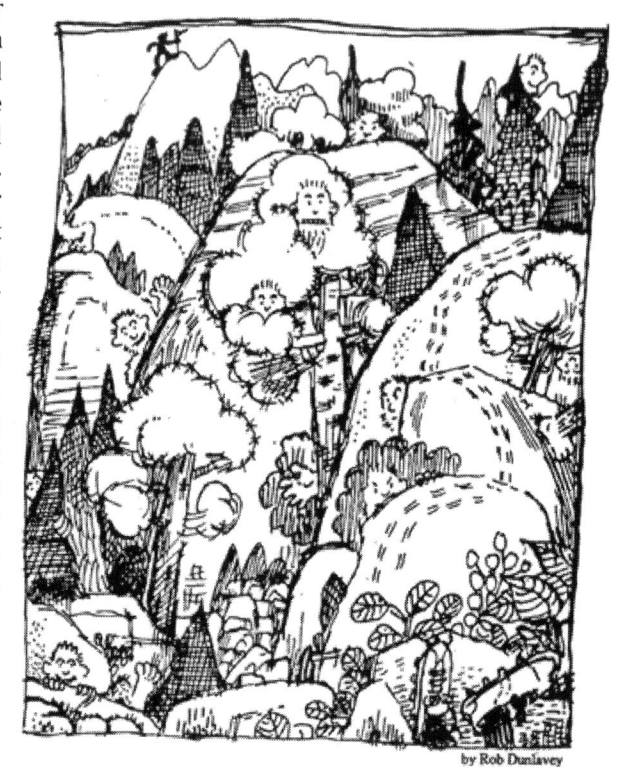

by Rob Dunlavey

body and his gear to Yakima Memorial Hospital. No report had come back yet from the coroner.

I asked Deputy Jones what she knew at this point. She said that she'd gone out with the first Search and Rescue Team, had seen the accident site and the body, and talked to a number of rogainers already. Several people confirmed that Phillips was an experienced orienteer, rogainer, and mountain climber. It looked as if he'd been killed by the 50-foot fall off the sandy cliff near the control location, but most rogainers she talked with seemed troubled: they doubted that he'd just slipped. Deputy Jones had found Phillips' prescription sunglasses next to the body. She was surprised that they were unbroken, considering what his face looked like. She had no evidence or information other than that. Deputy Jones did admit turning away and throwing up upon viewing the body.

Landchild told us that one of the staff had made a swing through the parking area and the adjacent road turnoffs right at 11 AM, recording license numbers of all cars in the area. It matched up exactly with the registration list and sign-in list. So he thinks that anyone that might have been on Spiral Butte around 10 AM was among our competitors, and on the Spiral Butte Intention Sheet. All rogaine event staff members were at a meeting in the Hash House area at 10 AM, so could not have been anywhere near the Spiral Butte summit between 8 AM and noon. I asked him about Phillips's car. He said he'd already checked on that. Phillips had ridden with Fulton in Fulton's new Mazda pickup. Fulton said that Phillips had no spare gear in his truck, except a box of cookies.

5:45 PM. I asked to talk to Phillips' partner, Wyatt Fulton next. I also asked all rogainers still present to remain at the campground until my partner and I could ask them questions about their knowledge of what happened. Fulton said, "I don't know what could have happened. Knut and I were having our best rogaine yet, had gotten all the controls, and were heading in to the Hash House about 10 AM this morning. We'd signed in at the last control at Spiral Butte, and I went ahead to scout the best route down. The only route choices were a dangerously steep scree slope, or further on to a steep, but passable forested slope. Either way there was a 1700-foot descent down the infant volcano's side, then a marsh to traverse.

"I chose the latter, and yelled back to him that I'd found a way, and was ready to descend. I heard a yell and heard him say 'I'm sliding down, meet you at the bottom.' So I slid on down some 1000 feet, then picked my way through the trees. I couldn't see or hear him, and he didn't answer my yells or whistle—but I know sounds don't carry far in the forest. Since we were very short on time, I figured he was trying to find his own way around Dog Lake to the finish. That's all I know—except that they'd found his body part-way down. I was asleep in my tent this afternoon when they took the body to Yakima."

Carl asked, "Did you see anyone near you on Spiral Butte?" Fulton said, "I can't be sure, but I thought I did get a glimpse of Scott MacDonald running along the trail to the lookout point, after I left Knut there. I was off-trail in the trees then, and couldn't see much except Scott's red hat. I remember that hat from

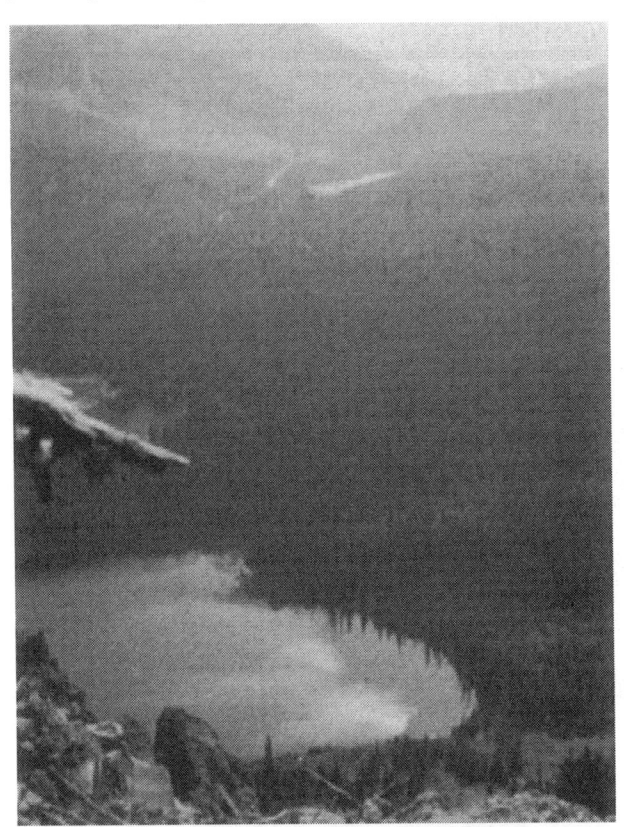

Dog Lake from the control #104 on top of Spiral Butte—the last 1 km leg, with a 1700-ft drop.

our earlier meeting at the waterfall. Come to think of it, Scott and Knut did look an awful lot alike—same build, age, and even the hat color. It could have been Knut, but he wouldn't have been going that way."

I asked, "Anything else?" Fulton replied, "Knut told me about a supposed fatal illness he'd just had diagnosed by some flaky doctor. Said he broke up with Kim Stark over it, and implied several times that this was his last rogaine. I felt pretty sure he was just exaggerating a minor complaint, which he often did. Now I'm not so sure."

I told Carl to call the hospital and get Murray Pugh, the coroner, a close associate, to give us a preliminary report on the deceased.

6:00 PM. We met with Miss Kim Stark of Team #22. She told us that she was a former girlfriend of Phillips, and they had lived together for several years. She said, "I was broken up when he told me that he'd acquired a fatal illness, had only a few months to go, and that I should move on and find someone else. I cried for a whole month. He was all I had, and I was all he had."

Then she told us her current teammate, Kent Ellsworth, was her new boyfriend. She said that both she and Phillips had told many of their rogaining friends about why they had broken up, and Knut knew about her new partner. She was going on about how Ellsworth was not as big and strong as Phillips, knew nothing about rogaining, but was so much more romantic, and sexier. I interrupted her to say, "Just the facts, Ma'am."

Miss Stark said she had not seen Phillips while they were on Spiral Butte, but she had been shocked speechless when she heard some noise on the trail behind her as they left Spiral Butte. She had glimpsed a large hairy, shadowy shape about 30 meters behind her just leaving the trail. Miss Stark tried to call out to her partner to look, but she couldn't get out a sound, and by then it was gone. She said, "I meant to tell Les Petty about what I thought I saw, but I haven't yet."

I asked, "Why tell Les Petty?" She said that she knew that Petty had been searching for signs of Bigfoot for over 20 years, from Northern California to British Columbia. He had never reported seeing anything but bogus footprints, and only heard a bunch of tall stories. Asked to describe her sighting further, she could provide nothing more, except that it seemed to move very fast and was over 8 feet tall, based on the lower branches of trees they had just passed under. She also commented that there was a terrible, putrid odor like burnt hair in the air.

Team #3, Peter Waugh and Fred Hudson, told us that they'd first met up with Team #13, Phillips and Fulton, at the waterfall about dawn, where they also saw Team #1. While refilling water bottles there, Phillips had pulled out a rock to make a deeper spot for his filter in the water. He discovered a curious partial jawbone under it. He showed it to his partner, and to the Team #3 and Team #1 members. Dr. MacDonald, an anthropologist from Washington State University, spent some time examining it closely. When he gave it back to Phillips, he said something about not tossing it away—it could be of some value. When Phillips asked why, MacDonald said that it looked like a jawbone of a large grizzly. He said there are only about 1000 grizzlies in the U. S., and they don't usually range this far south in the Cascades. He noted the bone also had teeth and a shape like a large ape, which might make it pre-Ice Age. By then the teams had finished water refilling, so conversation ended Phillips tucked the jawbone in under his belt above his rear pocket and went on.

Waugh said they'd later seen Team #13 at the Dancing Lady Lake control, but not on Spiral Butte, and not enroute back to the Hash House. Hudson remembered Phillips bragging that they'd got 54 controls.

We talked to Kent Ellsworth of Team #22 in the back of his dusty old Tercel station wagon. He was laid up with bad blisters, a serious sunburn, and a bad headache. Miss Stark was there bandaging him up, putting on sunburn ointment, and strapping on an ice pack. She explained that this was Ellsworth's first rogaine. We asked her to return to the Hash House tent while we questioned him. He stated that he had seen Phillips' partner Fulton briefly just after leaving Spiral Butte, but only at a distance. He didn't think Miss Stark saw Fulton. Nor did they linger in the area, as they thought they might be late getting back. As it was, they were late by some 50 minutes.

I asked Ellsworth about his occupation. He said he was an insurance salesman in Phillips' home town. Asked if he'd ever sold Phillips any insurance, he replied "no" after a long pause. Sensing an evasive answer, I immediately read him his rights, then probed his insurance sales. I warned him that the D.A. could subpoena all policies he had written, and that he could be prosecuted for lying, even if not directly involved. He then stated that he had sold a life insurance policy to Miss Stark, on Phillips's life. Miss Stark was the beneficiary. When asked if it had double indemnity for accidental death, he said yes, as was usual for such policies. I asked if it included a clause excluding suicide. Ellsworth said that it had the usual 6-month exclusion, but the policy was now seven months old. He was not willing to state the amount without a court order, but volunteered that it was the largest one he had ever written in his career. I asked about the 'fatal illness,' and when that had been diagnosed. He said all he knew was that Phillips had told him of an exam done about two months ago. The doctor thought there was a possibility of stomach cancer, but did not rule out less-serious ulcers.

Ellsworth stated that Miss Stark had never separated from him during the event, except for those few times when they went off for a "call of nature." [Note: Since this publication fails to qualify for placement at supermarket checkout newsracks, the gratuitous sex scenes you readers have been expecting or dreading have been omitted.] "Did you separate near Spiral Butte?" I asked. He said he couldn't remember. But he did remember something else. "What was that?" I inquired. He said, "I heard an eerie, high-pitched cry—sounded like a woman in trouble—I remember now—Kim was not in sight. I thought that she had injured herself. Yeah, it was just after we had left the Spiral Butte control. But she reappeared in a couple of minutes behind me, coming down the trail from the Spiral Butte lookout, and was OK. I remember asking if she'd heard the strange noise, but Kim seemed tongue-tied and kind of knackered, so I didn't ask again. We didn't hear it again, so I guess I forgot about it." Carl was taking notes. He asked, "What's 'knackered' mean?" Ellsworth replied, "Beats me. Some obscure term orienteers and rogainers use—something about dead horses, I think."

As we left for the Hash House tent, I noticed Ellsworth's muddy boots drying out on the hood of his car. Just then a rogainer walked by. Carl asked him who he was, and he introduced himself as Les Petty. We said we'd like to talk to him soon back at the Hash House tent. He just stood there a moment, looking all around, a frown on his face. Then he walked off without a word, heading through the parking area toward the outhouse. We noticed him writing something down in a notebook when he was almost out of sight.

DUM DE DUM DUM, DUMMMM.

PART II – Muddy Boots, a Curious Control Card – and Shakespeare!

The story continues. There'd been an accident during a rogaine and a man was dead. Detectives Sgt. Joe NotFriday and Officer Carl Newson are investigating.

DUM DE DUM DUM, DUM DE DUM DUM, DUMMMM. *(You have to be humming out loud, remember?)*

6:15 PM. Mr. Landchild told us that one of the staff had made a swing through the parking area and the adjacent road turnoffs right at 11 AM, recording license numbers of all cars in the area. It matched up exactly with the registration list and sign-in list. So he thinks that anyone that might have been on Spiral Butte around 10:00 AM was among our competitors, and on the Spiral Butte intention sheet. All rogaine event staff members were at a meeting in the Hash House area at 10 AM, so could not have been anywhere near Spiral Butte summit between 8 AM and noon. I asked him about Phillips's car. He said he'd already checked on that. Knut had ridden with Fulton in Wyatt's new Mazda pickup, and Wyatt said that Phillips had no spare gear in his truck, except a box of cookies.

I was curious about the muddy boots I'd just seen, since it seemed the entire area, except for the many small lakes, was bone dry this time of year. Landchild said he'd wondered also, having noticed that the last finishers had all come in with mud up to their ankles. He'd asked MacDonald, who told him that the teams coming down from Spiral Butte had all hit the marshy ground north of Dog Lake. They all had to go through it or around it, and cross two small streams to get back. His tent floor was covered with muddy tracks where those teams had come to log in.

6:30 PM. We saw Les Petty of Team #1 still nosing around the campground. We sat him down in the Hash House tent to question him. He told us that the only time he and MacDonald had seen Team #13 on the course was at a waterfall at about 6 AM Sunday. Team #3 was also there, very briefly. They had found Fulton and Phillips filling their water bottles from the stream at the foot of the falls, and he and MacDonald stopped to do the same. I asked if they talked about the rogaine, or exchanged route information. He said (expletive deleted or XD) no, as that was strictly against the rules. He strongly objected to all the questions with a few swear words thrown in for emphasis.

Disregarding Petty's objections and manner, I probed further about what happened there. At first he was surly and denied any knowledge of anything else. Finally he offered, "Yeah, there was one thing. We saw (XD) Knut pick up something from in the stream bed. He looked it over, and my partner went over to have a look, too. I saw it only from a distance. It looked like a (XD) piece of a jawbone of some large (XD) animal. MacDonald told Knut that he should not throw it away, as it was either a grizzly's jawbone, or perhaps that of an ape. If a bear, it was a kind not native to this area, and if an ape, it would be pre-Ice Age, and a rare find. We watched that (XD, XD) Knut tuck it under his belt on his left hip. I thought my (XD) partner would fill me in on it as we moved out to the next control. I knew he was an anthropologist at Mooo U (he meant WSU– Washington State University), and considered himself one of the world's top (XD) experts on bones. But Scott didn't bring up the subject, so I almost forgot about it."

Petty paused and sat quietly with his head down. I thought he might be dozing off with fatigue after the 24 hours on the course. But he resumed in a minute, with far fewer swear words, "I also recall, we did change our route plan right about then. Scott wanted to pick up a few more difficult controls over toward Dancing Lady Lake. I was surprised, since I thought he was about beat, but I agreed. He really picked up the pace then, walking way ahead of me so we couldn't talk. I thought I'd made him mad about something. Then I saw what MacDonald was up to. We'd been talking about the subtleties of navigation, wildlife and the wilderness area, taxa and the possibilities of many yet undiscovered species as well as the worldwide extinction of tens of thousands more each year. He loved to speculate on the worldwide fame that might come to a researcher who might discover a new species, or an old artifact that might add to scientific knowledge. We covered many other subjects over those first 18 hours,

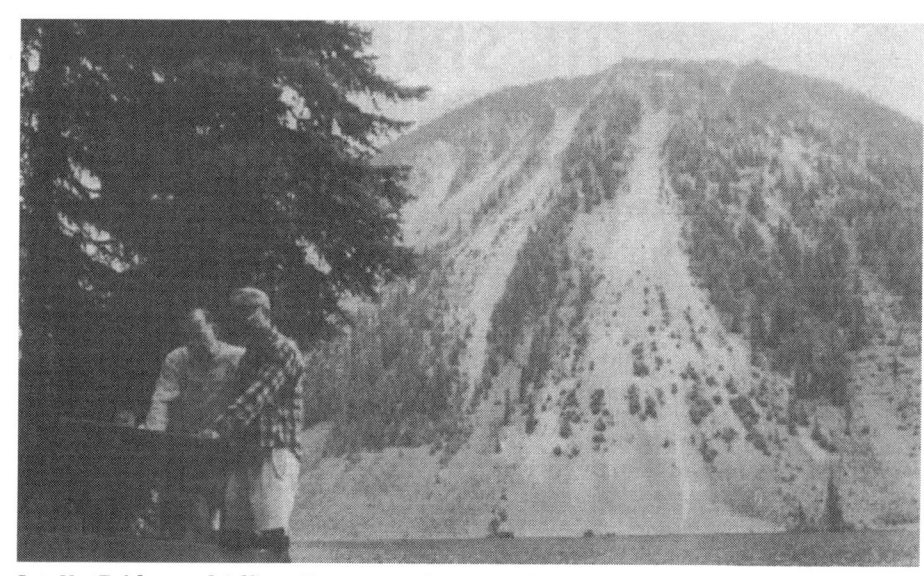

Sgt. NotFriday and Officer Newson at the Dog Lake Campground below Spiral Butte.

8

so I was really (XD) (he meant 'upset') when Scott clammed up and started walking ahead. This partnership and friendly teamwork aspect of rogaining was the main reason I took up this sport. I've really enjoyed this rogaining, even though I've rarely won anything in the Masters' Class."

I asked Petty what he meant when he said, "Then I saw what he was up to." He just stared at the floor. I repeated my question, but again he didn't respond.

Suddenly Petty looked up and retorted, "I'm not helping you lousy (XD) coppers any more. I'm a Canadian citizen, and you can't touch me without charges." I asked what his occupation was. He turned very nasty then, and said he'd need to talk to his lawyer first, if I needed anything else.

7:00 PM. I next interviewed Dr. Scott MacDonald of Team #1. He told me pretty much what his partner had said about MacDonald's position at WSU, and their meeting Team #13 and Team #3 at the waterfall. He said the bone was most likely a bear, and that it was very rare to find any kind of big wild animal bone in the forest, since Mother Nature so quickly recycled them. I inquired about his partner, Mr. Petty. He said it was the first time he had rogained with him. He said that Petty seemed to be an excellent navigator, probably due to his extensive guide work, hunting and man-tracking experience. He also said Petty struck him as a crafty and scheming type, somewhat moody, and had a 'Nixonian' style of speech. I asked if he or Petty had seen either Fulton or Phillips after leaving the waterfall. He then stated that he would have to consult with his lawyer if I had any more questions, and after that said nothing further. I reminded him not to leave the area, and then told Carl to have Deputy Linda Jones keep an eye on him.

7:10 PM. Carl said, "Here's what's happening. I got a call from Coroner Pugh. He is faxing the documents found to us. Phillips' death was instantaneous, due to a massive blow to the head There were minor cuts, mosquito bites, and bruises also, some of which may have come from the fall. He said a complete report will come when the autopsy is done. Phillips' pack had an old patch sewn to the top flap that says: "Rogaine USA '89, First Place". The pack contained the usual essentials: pen, knife, matches, extra eyeglasses, two PowerBars, small Rite-in-the-Rain notebook with "Knut Phillips" written on the cover—no entries in it, toothbrush, toilet paper, compass, windbreaker jacket, rain hood, rain pants, two water bottles (one empty), a partly used packet of Gookinaid, water pump and filter, small flashlight (batteries dead), and two good batteries. In a first aid kit cover were a spare bulb, insect repellent stick, tw0 bandaids, one piece of moleskin, tiny scissors, and some dental floss. In this kit also were some prescription pills that the coroner recognized as a painkiller for those in the final stages of a fast acting cancer. His Silva compass was tied to his right wrist. A Toyota key was threaded on his right bootlace and tucked under one gaiter. There was no map, no regular punch card, nor the animal bone you asked about on him. There was a card with written entries on it, but no punches. There was also a small nylon wallet containing $25 cash, his driver's license with photo, and his telephone credit card, and a card handwritten in the same way as his signature as follows:

> To die – to sleep –
> No more; – and, by a sleep, to say we end
> The heart-ache, and the thousand natural shocks,
> That flesh is heir to, – 'Tis a consummation
> Devoutly to be wish'd
>
>   Shakespeare.

Carl said, "Joe we've got a problem."
"What's that, Carl?"
"Too many suspects! "
"Yeah! Go over the list again?"

"Sure. Here goes:
1. Knut Phillips, himself–a possible suicide, anticipating painful final days of illness.
2. Wyatt Fulton, Knut Phillips' partner– the partners argued over something, or a mercy killing?
3. Scott MacDonald, the anthropologist– he gets bone, with worldwide fame and maybe fortune.
4. Les Petty, MacDonald's partner– knows something, but not talking. He wanted the bone, too?
5. Kim Stark, the ex-girlfriend beneficiary of big insurance policy, or revenge over the breakup with Phillips. She may have figured his news of his fatal illness was just a ploy to dump her.
6. Kent Ellsworth, the insurance agent– double indemnity payoff, if he's in it with Miss Stark.
7. Peter Waugh –eliminate the competition, get K*Swiss deal.
8. Fred Hudson–same as Waugh; get other team out of it and win.
9. How about this one, Joe–the Sasquatch! Phillips desecrated a grave and took a relative's bone, or maybe it's Bigfoot mating season and he looked like competition. Ha!
10. And how about just a slip and fall–a tired man admiring Mt. Rainier?

"Too many possibilities, Joe! At least ten, maybe more–if you count some conspiracies in there."

"Carl, you're right. Let's look over the event results and those time sheets—what're they called? intention sheets?—again. Can we tell anything about this 'quest' of rogainers—their locations and movements around Dancing Lady Lake and Spiral Butte where Phillips was last seen and heard? I've already puzzled over them, and they don't tell me much, except every one of these four rogaine teams was close by. Anyone could have falsified their entries on the log sheets, I suppose. But to what purpose? No one has reported anything unusual about these entries when we had each person review those log sheets. Wait a minute! We've gotten the fax of this curious second control card now. Let's talk to Team #3 about it."

7:15 PM. I talked to Team #3 member Peter Waugh. I asked, "Mr. Waugh, at an early control, Knut Phillips was seen copying something off the intention sheet onto a card (it looked like his punch card). The coroner found in his pack a card with "X" entries in several blocks (not punches). Here's a faxed copy of this curious card. In the Total column you'll see he entered #3, then 21, 22, 23, 25, 26, 42,–49, 31, 61, 44, 51, 24, 52, 33, 101, etc. Mean anything to you?" Waugh stated that this was the order in which his team visited those controls.

Fred Hudson, Waugh's partner, joined us at my request. I showed him the fax of this strange control card, then asked them both how Mr. Phillips could have determined their team route and made these entries during the event Waugh speculated that Phillips must have looked at the intention sheet at each control, noted whether Team #3 had already been there, plus their time of arrival and where they were going next. If Team #13 had been following them, or by coincidence taking exactly the same route or order of visit to the controls, then this should be a complete log of Team #3's rogaine control visits. However, he pointed out, this list was incomplete. Hudson said, "I knew from seeing intention sheets during the event that Team #13 had reached some controls before we did. We had only sighted Team #13 at a distance in several scattered parts of the rogaine area on Saturday. We knew it was "Big-Foot" Phillips (we called him that sometimes because of his size 16 feet) from his red hat. Sunday, we had seen them only at the waterfall and Dancing Lady Lake while punching in."

Peter Waugh observed, "Veerrrry in-ter-es-ting! It isn't clear to me why "Big-Foot" Phillips was doing this recording, but I'm suspicious. Maybe he was just curious about our route—but this would have been revealed to all after the finish, and probably published in the final results report in a month or two. To try to obtain this while actually competing in a timed event seems very peculiar. In previous competitions,

I had seen, and later confirmed with Knut and his partner, that their standard rogaining routine at each control went like this: Wyatt would quickly sign the intention sheet, then move off about 100 meters in the direction of the next control. He did almost all the team's compass work and initial route planning, since Knut never did like using a compass, and almost never used one. Then he'd stop, drink water, and study the map in a place that would not reveal the just-left control's location to other approaching teams. Meanwhile, Knut would log in, punch the team's single control card, and then sit down there and take a quick break for map-reading, food, and water.

"So Knut was always alone at each control for 1 to 5 minutes. Many others who competitively rogained knew of this somewhat aberrant team procedure. Competitors often questioned organizers whether this was violating the rule that team members must stick together. Knut and Wyatt were previously let go with just warnings, as it was concluded that no competitive advantage was being obtained. Since each team member knew that his partner was stopped close by, no safety degradation was evident, either."

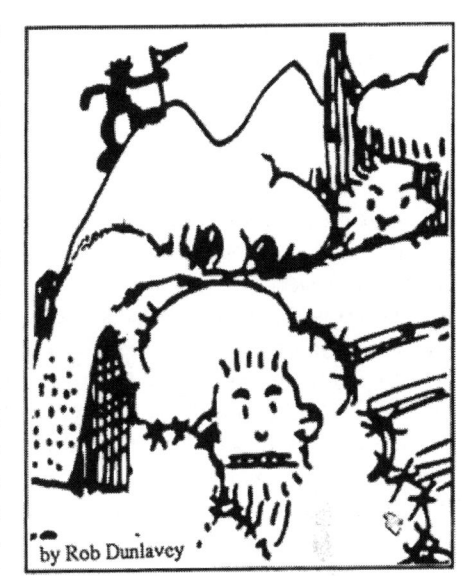

I thought, "Not in this case—to the contrary!"

Mr. Hudson then interrupted, "Something just struck me! Remember that control we couldn't locate at 2 AM Sunday morning? (He paused for effect, leaving Carl and me waiting for something useful).

DUM DE DUM DUM–DUM DE DUM DUM, DUMMMM.

PART III – The Jawbone, the Rock, and the Confessional!

The story continues. There'd been an accident during a rogaine and a man was dead. Detectives Sgt. Joe NotFriday and Officer Carl Newson are investigating. They were questioning team #3, Peter Waugh and Fred Hudson, when Hudson remembers something.

DUM DE DUM DUM, DUM DE DUM DUM, DUMMMM. *(You have to be humming out loud, remember?)*

Fred Hudson then interrupted, "Something just struck me! Remember that control we couldn't locate at 2 AM Sunday morning? We searched back and forth around those three meadows and didn't find the control. I asked Kalon Stradeski of Team #6 about it. He told me they found that control bag just after daylight, about 6 AM, and were lucky to spot it. It was tangled up in a tree branch on a single tree in the middle of the largest of those three meadows. The bag was collapsed so that the reflective tape was not detectable by a flashlight, and even the intention sheet was tangled around the branch. Kalon said he noted that Team #13 had been there at about 1 AM, and most likely couldn't have found it either, if it had been like that then. So Kalon guessed that an animal had pulled at it during the night. There were footprints of enormous size all around it."

I asked, "Did he say 'footprints', or 'hoofprints'?" Hudson guessed that Stradeski meant animal tracks. I asked to talk to Stradeski, but he'd already left for his home in California. Fred Hudson went on to say, "We found one control ourselves which had been pulled down and trampled on earlier on Saturday. But it was an easy location to find, so we rehung the control and moved on. But now, I'm wondering if Team #13, either Knut or Wyatt, might have tampered with that control? And the others we had trouble with? I don't want to speak ill of the dead, but with the potential sponsorship by K*Swiss of the winning team from this event, and maybe big endorsement and travel money...? (his voice trailed off). Team #13 had won the very first rogaine in the US back in 1989, then had come in second to our team in five other rogaines, always just a few points behind. Both Wyatt Fulton and "Big-Foot" Phillips were Type A, hotly competitive types, who were always goading each other on to their endurance limits. Both Phillips and Fulton would often get really angry and throw things around when events didn't go their way. Peter and I used to say that they were "over-torqueing" this sport—but then, we've been accused of the same. We even used that disparaging word jokingly for the name of our team for this event. We were always trying to find ways to obtain a competitive advantage to be sure to beat them. We spent many hours running up steep hillsides, and even bought these backpack water bladders with the drinking tubes to minimize our water stops. We are exceptionally good at selecting optimum routes to minimize climb. In reviewing event results, I found that the routes of Knut and Wyatt were very much like ours, but usually included one or two controls that were just not 'gettable' by them within the time constraint. So they often lost on penalty points."

I asked if he meant that they often bit off more than they could chew. Waugh said yes, and that they were surprised to hear Phillips tell them at Dancing Lady Lake that Team #13 had gotten 54 controls so far, and were going for their last one. Hudson saw on the Dancing Lady Lake Intention Sheet that Team #13 was going for the Spiral Butte control, where they were also headed.

Waugh said, "We could see by the map that it was a very tough climb up, and perhaps an even harder descent to get back to the Hash House before the 12 noon deadline. We calculated that we still had a chance to beat Team #13. And we were still feeling very fit. We ate a PowerBar each and moved out. Considering the remaining time, it looked like any team going for Spiral Butte from here would find it almost impossible to get back to the finish on time. With a 10-point-per-minute penalty for being late, our team's 80-point deficit (two controls missed) would be offset by another team arriving just 8 or more minutes late and later than us. So we went hard for Spiral Butte, and took a fairly chancy sliding route down the steep west side. As it turned out, we were two minutes late getting back. We didn't see Team #13 again after leaving Dancing Lady."

At this point I took Waugh aside and asked him about his movements to and around Spiral Butte. He said they had seen Phillips and Fulton by Dancing Lady Lake, noted that they were going to Spiral Butte also, but didn't see them going up there. He said, "We got to the control pretty fast, and saw by the log that they hadn't arrived. We then split up to try to find the quickest safe route down. I went north, and Fred went southeast from the lookout point. After about five minutes or so, Fred and I met as agreed. He said there was no way down back there, so we went down the northwestern slope where I'd been scouting. That's about it—we didn't see or hear Team #13 at all." I asked if Hudson's search might have brought him back past the control again. He conceded that it was possible.

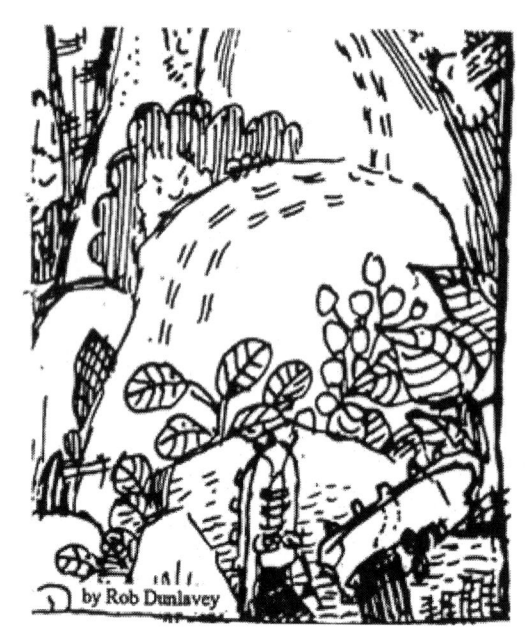

7:25 PM. Landchild brought over two pieces of paper that some of his staff had found while recovering controls. The first was the missing control card for Team #13, showing five blocks with punches in them. He pointed out that this was the card that the deceased should have had on him when he fell. But this had been found near a control where that team had been early on the first day. The second paper was a rogaine map, with no identification on it. But there was something unusual about it. Landchild showed me that at many of the control locations on the map, there were holes obviously made by the

by Rob Dunlavey

control location punches. The punches had been made right on top of the marked control location circles. He had immediately suspected that this was the missing map of Team #13. It had been found about half way between Dancing Lady Lake and Spiral Butte, in brush on a steep slope in the forest. He had counted the punches—there were 49. He checked the six unpunched controls, and found that five were the ones punched on the just-found control card. All were there except #104, Spiral Butte, which was not punched on either the card or the map.

I asked Landchild what he made of these papers and the punches. He explained the rule that the punch card was the primary proof of a team's visit to controls, and that team results and scores were calculated based on the card. Damage or loss of the control card was cause for disqualification, unless the team could somehow show or prove beyond doubt that they had visited each control claimed. The intention sheets were never used for this purpose, since they were often not all recovered in legible shape. He said, "Some were often damaged by animals, and we didn't expect to get them all in until days or weeks after the event. I thought that the punches in the map were Knut's method of recording them, having apparently lost the control card early in the event, and too far from the base camp to get another. He was probably hoping that this card would be found, or that they would outscore other teams even without the five 20-pointer controls recorded on it. Losing the map, though, put them out of the event altogether. It was sheer luck that it was found at all in that thick brush."

I asked Landchild about the curious second control card. He said Phillips must have picked up an extra card when he registered Saturday morning. He noted that Phillips could have used it when he lost the other one, but obviously he was using it for something else, so punched on the map instead. He didn't want to speculate on the card's entries or use. None of this punch stuff seemed relevant to the case, so I told Carl to file these papers in our briefcase.

7:45 PM. Carl summarized, "Here's what we've got, Joe. It's not much, or maybe it's too much! All our searching so far hasn't turned up the missing bone fragment. We still have one or two deputies up there on Spiral Butte searching. That card in Phillips' wallet isn't the usual kind of suicide note that we sometimes find. We don't know for sure if he really had a fatal illness until we can trace down his doctor. That girl Kim and the insurance bozo Kent are both acting nervous as hell. "XD" (expletive deleted) Petty has gone off to sulk about something. That anthropologist guy MacDonald seems extremely quiet, and looks devastated—and he'd never met Phillips before this event, so he says. I don't believe in all those Bigfoot tales, but I've heard them from my grandfather and from Indian tribal members around the Cascades here all my life. They've told me that the Sasquatch is mostly a nocturnal creature, and very reclusive. Sightings by Indians and backwoods people are extremely rare, a tiny percentage of bear sightings, which are rare enough. That winning team, Waugh and Hudson, seem not to be elated over their victory. Wonder if it's because they know that they would have been beaten, if not for this mishap. Or maybe the notoriety of the outcome of this event may kill their chances of a big sponsor endorsement. Fulton seems doubly shocked that he lost both his partner and winning this event at the very last control. I wonder when or if he knew that their punch card was lost. Was he helping Knut tamper with controls? And, don't forget, this still could be just an accidental fall."

Carl said, "Our Mobile Crime Lab artist, Margie York, drew up this sketch of the jawbone. Waugh, Fulton, and Hudson gave her ideas, and said it's a good likeness. But MacDonald and Petty had no comments. They're pretty cagey about this bone deal."

"This is giving me a headache, Carl. Let's take a break for some coffee and a smoke."

"Suits me, Joe. There's some coffee on over by the campfire."

7:55 PM. The rogaine caterer, Jane Verbeck, greeted us and said she still had a hot dog or two and some fruit left over. "Brown-eyed Jane", as everyone called her, told us she'd packed up and was ready to leave for home at Nelson Siding, when she'd heard of the accident, and saw several people were staying. She told us that the participants had consumed most all of the $1500 in food, but that she'd saved enough for the late returnees, particularly those who hadn't returned to the Hash House for dinner or breakfast.

13

Everyone but Phillips had eaten by 1:30 PM, including the organizers. She had not talked to anyone in particular since then, but told us she had overheard Kim whispering with some man about a rock having been thrown at Knut. "Brown-eyed Jane" couldn't tell us who the man was, or anything else of value, but offered us the crumbs from a pan of carrot cake (my favorite) she'd forgotten she had, and had just served. She poured us two cups and I was ready to light up when we were interrupted.

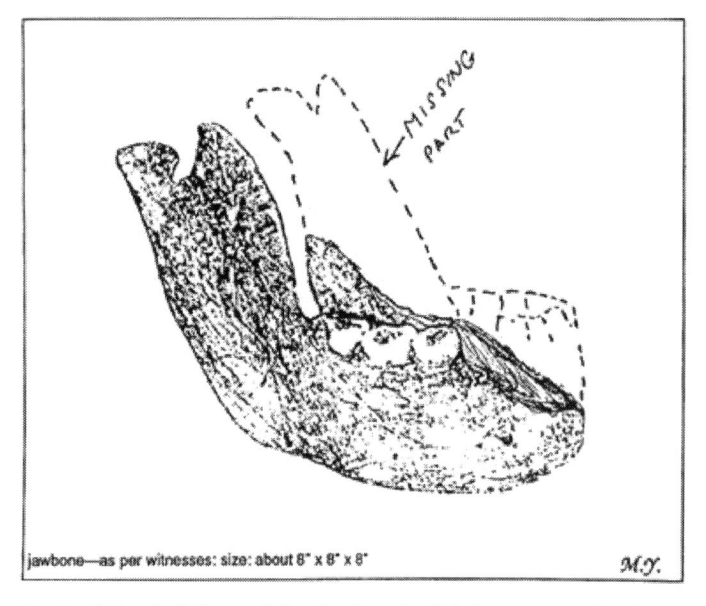

"Sgt. NotFriday, come take a look at this," said just-returned Deputy Sheriff Jan Skog, who'd been searching the cliff area. "What's that, Jan?" I responded. "It's a rock with blood on it, and probably Phillips' hair, Joe. Weighs about 7 1/2 pounds. Our Mobile Crime Lab (MCL) will confirm whose blood and hair. We've also been able to lift a fingerprint—looks like a big thumb—off this smooth area right here."

I asked, "Where'd you find this rock?" Skog said, "It was part way down the cliff, about one-half way to where the body was found. It was also off about 15 feet to the East of the fall line of the body—it didn't go straight down with him." I asked if he'd seen any sign of a jawbone, or anything else. He responded, "Yes, Deputy Good found this Leki hiking pole with his red hat on top, propped against a tree right at the edge of the 50-foot cliff." He handed them to me, and I looked both over. Nothing unusual about them, except that the pole had a spring-loaded shaft to absorb shock. I showed them to Fulton and he identified them as Phillips'.

Deputy Skog pointed out, "Match that fingerprint up with one of these rogainer's thumbs, and you've got your man!"

I thought to myself, "Or maybe a woman!"

TUM, TUM, TUM, TUM, TUM, TA-TA-TA, TUM *(A higher pitch, please—the plot thickens.)*

8:00 PM. Carl and I called everyone together around the campfire, and told them to sit down and wait. Then we took each rogainer separately over to a picnic table near the lake. Carl read each of them his/her rights and got affirmation that each understood. Then I asked each one the following question: "We've got the rock. Care to tell me about it before we put the cuffs on?" I dangled my handcuffs menacingly as each one answered, and sipped at my almost cold coffee.

Wyatt Fulton came back in a whimpering voice, "OK, sure I threw the rock. But I missed, and Knut didn't even see or hear it. He was right there on the edge of the cliff, and I thought he might just turn quickly and lose his balance in trying to see where it came from. It would have been a quick end to his painful final days of his illness—a mercy killing, you might say. I got so scared at what I'd almost done, that I ran on to the slope edge, and called back to him to come on quick. I heard him yell something about meeting me at the bottom,

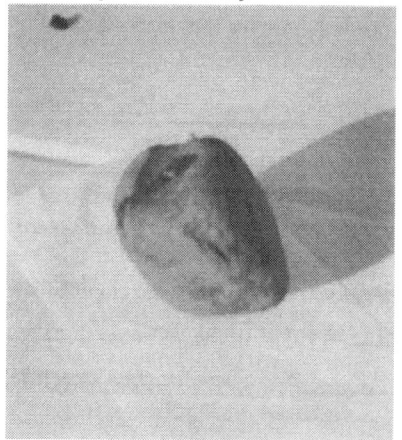

jawbone—as per witnesses: size: about 8" x 8" x 8"   M.J.

Rock with blood, hair, and tissue, and a large fingerprint.
Photo by G. Taylor, Y.P.D.

14

so I started the slide down to meet him there. I didn't want to say anything about the rock, since nothing had happened. I was outraged about his first losing the punch card, and then later the map with the rest of the punches, and for not telling me about it. I told him a million times to pin that punch card to his shirt. Too bad he fell, but I didn't do it!

"I also wonder if all this had anything to do with the note to him I found in my truck yesterday." I asked,

"What note?" Fulton dug into his pack and pulled out an envelope and unfolded it. He handed it to me and told me he had found it on the truck floor after Phillips had taken his pack out Saturday morning. I looked at the envelope. It had a logo for the N*Swoosh sports shoe company on it–they were the biggest competitor of K*Swiss. The note inside was typewritten on plain paper. It said: "Knut–confirming our call, do it as planned and we'll double their deal. R." I asked Fulton what he knew of this. He said he'd seen the note was to Knut, didn't know what it meant, and had planned to return it to him, but had put it into his pack and just remembered it while waiting for this interrogation. I thanked him, mulled this over for a minute, then called for the next rogainer.

Fred Hudson said forcefully, "OK, sure I threw the rock. But I missed, and Phillips didn't even see or hear it. He was standing right there on the bluff edge, and I thought he might just turn quickly and lose his balance in trying to see where it came from. It would have been a quick end to his painful illness. But I was just expecting to delay him if he was just dazed or scraped up in the fall–enough to cause him to get to the finish a few minutes late. I'd figured out that he'd been the one concealing those controls from my team so they'd win. I was in a blind rage! But I got so scared at what I'd almost done, that I ran back to rejoin my partner, and didn't say anything until now about it. I couldn't find Peter right away, and I was afraid he was back there going to try the same thing! But we got together in the next two minutes, and started our slide down. Too bad he fell, but I didn't do it!"

8:20 PM. My cellular phone rang, interrupting the interrogation. I prayed that it might be something helpful...

DUM DE DUM DUM, DUMMMM.

PART IV – Boomer, the Thumbprint Match, and the Sasquatch

The story continues. There'd been an accident during a rogaine and a man was found dead. The case is still unsolved. It's apparently a difficult one, but there are plenty of clues. You, dear reader, are undoubtedly much smarter than the investigating detectives Sgt. Joe NotFriday and Officer Carl Newson. Sgt. NotFriday hears his cellular phone. Read on...

DUM DE DUM DUM, DUM DE DUM DUM, DUMMMM. *(You are, by now, regularly humming out loud, aren't you?)*

8:20 PM. My cellular phone rang, interrupting the interrogation. I prayed that it might be something helpful. It was a call from Deputy Susan Miller of the SAR Search Team. She said she'd returned home to Naches after the body had been found, but had heard that we were doing a thorough accident investigation and wanted to report something. She reported that she and Boomer had arrived at about 3 PM Her dog had just been introduced to the lost person's scent in the Mazda when the report came in that the body had been found. She was relieved to hear the search was over, because her Golden Retriever had reacted very strangely to the scent in the truck. Boomer had shaken her head, yelped, ran back to her car, and jumped in through the open tailgate. Deputy Miller's efforts to cajole her to come out had finally succeeded just when the body was brought down from Spiral Butte and placed in the ambulance. As the body passed by, Boomer alerted, gave the same yelp, and jumped back in the car.

The deputy had rewarded the dog with her favorite rawhide bone treat anyway, then checked out with the SAR team chief and drove home. Miller said that the only time anything like this had happened before was when they'd encountered a skunk during a search. Boomer had learned the hard way not to tackle that kind of critter.

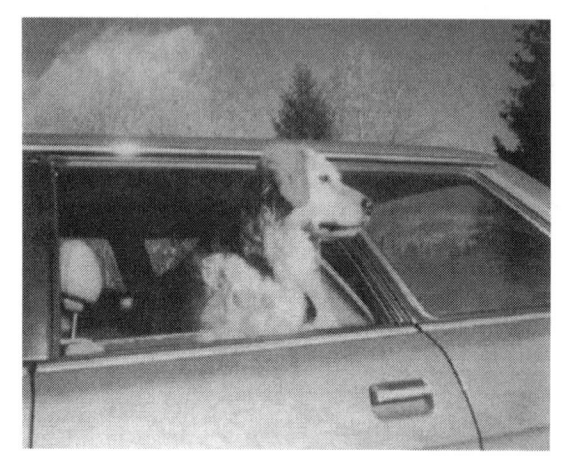

I thanked Miller for her report, and was ready to hang up when she said, "Wait, there's something else! As we were driving out of the parking lot after the ambulance had left, Boomer started acting up in the rear seat, and then nosed my ear for another treat. I scolded her to stop that while I was driving, and then I forgot about it. Boomer's still in training, and I don't know all her quirks well. But she's been good knowing when a reward is due. I thought you ought to know."

I thanked her again and we hung up. I told myself to remember to tell Carl later about the distressed, neurotic dog. My eye caught the N*Swoosh envelope I'd taken from Fulton. A stain was in the corner, so for some reason I sniffed it. My eyes immediately watered and I coughed hard. Smelled something like cat urine. I puzzled over this a moment, and thought that in this Spiral Butte case, "spiral" equals "convoluted" equals "screwed up." Even Spiral Butte itself was "sinister" or "sinistral," since it turns to the left. It seems that fate, Murphy's Law, or something sinister (in all its meanings) was turning this case into a massive misadventure.

8:27 PM. We resumed the questioning. Scott MacDonald admitted, "OK, sure I threw the rock. But I missed, and Knut didn't even react. He was right on the edge of the cliff, staring at that jawbone. I thought he might just turn quickly and lose his balance trying to see where it came from. It would have been a quick end to the final days of his painful illness. I was hoping he'd just drop the bone and forget it, and I could go back and pick it up later. Deputy Jones and I did search later, but with no luck. I got so scared at what I'd almost done that I ran back to rejoin my partner, and Les and I then went to the control and signed in. There was no sign of either Knut or Wyatt there, but I thought I heard someone sliding down the slope below us. I didn't say anything until now about the rock. Too bad he fell, but I didn't do it!" I sent him back to the campfire.

A thought struck me, and I asked Carl, "I know most of the deputies around here, but not Linda Jones. Is she new?" Carl said, "Yeah, she moved here about a month ago from Pullman. She was with the WSU Campus Police." I thought about that, then called for the next rogainer.

Kim Stark said about the same thing as the others: "OK, sure I threw the rock. But I missed, and my old flame didn't even see or hear it. He was there on the edge of the cliff when I came past while searching for a way down. I thought he might just turn quickly and lose his balance in trying to see where it came from. It would have been a merciful end to his painful final days with his fatal illness. I loved him so! I got so scared at what I'd almost done that I ran back to rejoin my partner, who was waiting for me down the trail. I didn't say anything about it to anyone until now. It's tragic that he fell, but I didn't do it!"

The other three—Peter Waugh, Les Petty, and Kent Ellsworth (we woke him up), refused to even respond to my rock question ploy, and demanded to talk to their attorneys first. Waugh seemed both nervous and dejected. Ellsworth was helpful in showing us his team's split time from Spiral Butte to the Hash House on his Casio. It showed (assumed 2 hrs.) 46:35.08 minutes. He said his blisters, the scree slope, and the muddy marsh really slowed them down. Petty said something about looking at tracks and strongly suggested that I remove my (XD=expletive deleted) head from an anatomically impossible position. Carl grabbed me as I was about to stimulate Petty into a nasty "accidental" fall against the picnic table with my stun gun.

9:00 PM. We lit a lantern. I exclaimed, "This doesn't compute, Carl! They've all got almost the same story. Four of them have admitted to attempted murder, or at least to a dangerous violent act, which could have led to a death. And they all have a motive, some not very provable, and certainly the opportunity! I need to get back to the vice, narcotics, and gambling beat–where things are more open-and-shut! Wait! I wonder if we should show them the rock and get their reactions?"

Carl said, "Yeah, let's try it." Carl separately asked each of the four admitted rock-throwers to look in the evidence box secured in our truck, while I watch their expressions. Each one immediately exclaimed, "That's not the rock! Too big!" The three men betrayed no other emotions. Stark broke down crying. I wanted to cry, too. We were getting nowhere. Carl added, "And don't forget Mt. Rainier! The mountain's not talking, but several people told me that the mountain was out on both days. But the only way to see it from Spiral Butte was to lean way out by the cliff edge to look at it. Knut could have just slipped on that sandy bluff edge trying to get a good look. Or urinating. And we already know it could be suicide—but then what would have been the point of trying so hard to win this event? Maybe even tampering with some controls to hamper other teams? Joe, do you think anyone's telling the whole truth?"

"Some are, some aren't, Carl. And maybe someone's covering up for someone else. There are lots of strange happenings and puzzles in this case. Too many rock-throwers. Landchild, Fulton, and Stark gave the SAR Team descriptions of Phillips clothing. They matched those on the deceased, according to the SAR people plus Landchild and Stark. The coroner told us on the phone that the clothing and boots were brand new, but the backpack was old.

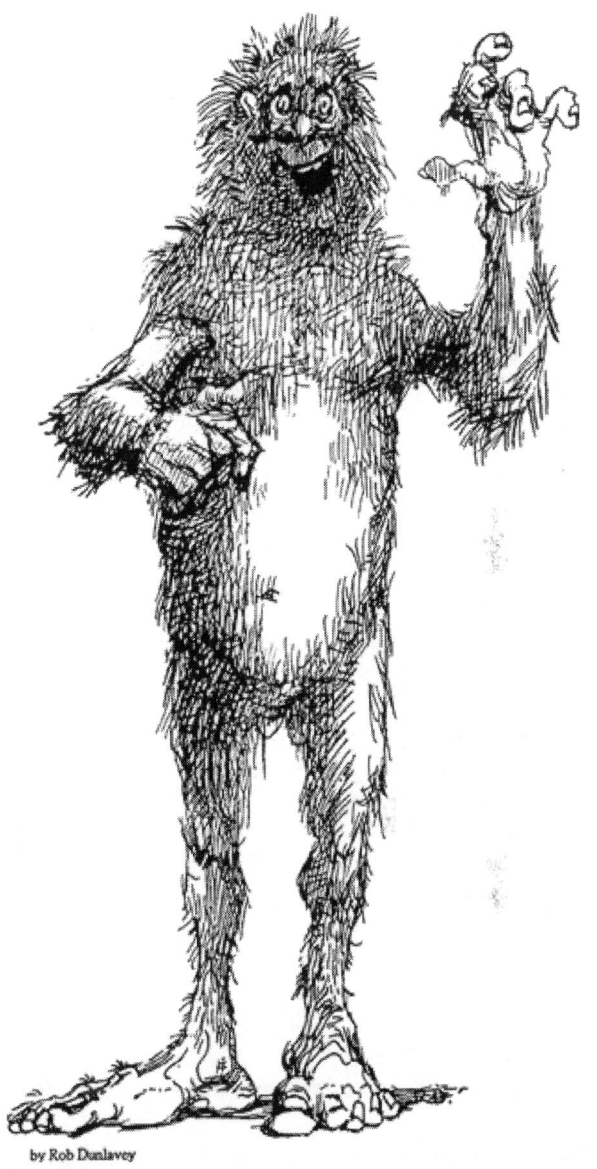

Carl inquired, "What bothers you about that, Joe?" I replied, "Carl, it seems strange to me that an experienced rogainer would wear new boots to a 24-hour rogaine. I've heard that some of these lightweight hiking boots from REI require little break-in, but it still seems peculiar. Also, what is it that Petty knows and won't reveal? Another thing—where's Phillips's wristwatch? The coroner didn't find it, and according to what Landchild told me, he was wearing a very expensive Rolex. Why on a rogaine? Fulton also saw it, but no one else remembered it."

Carl speculated, "It could have just come off in the fall. We'd probably never find a watch on that scree slope—we couldn't find the bone. Or, maybe someone stole it off the corpse."

I replied, "Yeah, maybe. You know, we had reports about tracks from the deputies up at the Spiral Butte lookout. They said there was a lot of ground disturbance there, but the soil was too firm to show up any identifiable footprints. He could have just fallen, but I think he probably had help. Big as he was, I still suspect someone or some thing probably pushed or threw him off. Or maybe they all did!"

I asked Carl to read out our suspect list one last time. He made it quick: "The Sasquatch, retaliation for the bone theft; a suicide—facing cancer, an accidental fall; Wyatt Fulton blows up, throws rock and fights partner—maybe accidentally knocks him off cliff, then grabs bone and watch; Kim Stark, woman scorned, insurance, too; Kent Ellsworth, pushed him over for payoff with or without Kim's knowledge; Peter Waugh, the rogaine win brings contract; Fred Hudson, nails Phillips for cheating; Scott MacDonald, in a struggle for bone, Phillips slipped or pushed; Les Petty, maybe helped MacDonald or went for bone himself; and last, perhaps several of them.

"Never saw anything as screwy as this case, Joe! Add in that 'hair-covered thing' sighting to twist it further! It's too bad there were no Sasquatch footprints found anywhere around. That volcanic-ash, sandy cliff bank edge was stirred up, all right. But we have no concrete evidence. You can't go into court with a 'nasty smell' or an 'eerie high-pitched scream.' Not like the old days, Joe."

"How's that, Carl?"

"We always solved these cases in a half hour!"

9:30 PM. It was really dark. Just then everyone was startled by a loud cry coming from high up on Spiral Butte. The sound made the hairs on the back of my neck stand up. Deputy Skog's radio squawked, and he got a call. He reported the conversation to me. Said it was Deputy K. E. Greenlee (or Keg, they called him), searching around up at the scene of the fall, who was just wrapping up for the night. Seems someone, or some thing just threw a big rock at Keg, and he was coming back down the fastest way he could find. Keg also wanted to have the word passed to the Sheriff Enger that he is going back home to Yakima and wouldn't be coming up this way again, ever!

9:40 PM. Carl and I looked across the lake and could just make out a headlamp of someone—it had to be Keg—coming down the Spiral Butte slope in the dark, very fast. Carl and I looked at each other. We then assembled the so-called "quest" of rogainers, and I announced that just as soon as we finger-printed everyone who'd volunteer at our MCL in the campground parking lot, and got their addresses, we'd be releasing them to go home. We'd let them know if anything further was needed after the lab work on the rock was done. I said anyone not wanting to be printed or give information would be driven to Yakima tonight for a stay in our 80-year-old, non-air-conditioned city jail–while we thought up some more questions. I was not surprised when they all agreed to prints. Our specialist even woke up Ellsworth again to get his.

As we packed up and were starting to scatter to our cars, Carl's cellular phone rang. It was Sgt. Graham Taylor at the Mobile Crime Lab with a preliminary report. Carl said, "Joe, you're not going to like this."

"Yeah, how's that?"

'The blood and the tissue on the rock are not human. The hair is not from Phillips but from some unidentified animal. The lab analyst, Dave Sharp, thinks it's possibly a skunk—bad stench on the rock. And the fingerprint on the rock–yeah, the very last set Graham checked—it matched a thumbprint from the hiking stick and the right thumb of—(I hate it when he pauses like that)—guess who?"

"Spit it out, Carl."

"The deceased!"

10:00 PM. We got in the Land Cruiser and headed back. While driving and thinking for a few miles I said, "Carl, here's what we'll do. File this case as unsolved. Let the insurance investigator on the multi-million-dollar accidental death claim work it. I think we might've missed the key to this case, but maybe it'll eventually turn up. Or maybe another detective, reading our report, will hit on the solution."

Carl objected, "But, Joe! You've never bagged a case before." I concluded, "Yeah, but we've never run up against a Sasquatch before, and I sure don't want to meet this one. Kind of ironic, don't you think, Carl?"

"How's that, Joe?"

"Bigfoot killed 'Big-Foot'!"

DUM DE DUM DUM, DUMMMM.

The Yakima County DA reviewed the case and agreed to file it as unsolved. The coroner found serious ulcers but no cancer in the body's stomach. Local fingerprint checks produced nothing, and the FBI results will take months. The insurance company is going to have to pay up on the $2.5 million policy to Stark if they don't get some fresh leads for their investigation. They have nothing solid to support a suicide or murder finding. It'll cost them $5 million if they blame it on the Sasquatch or call it an accident. Rumor is that they do not intend to accept the existence of the Sasquatch. The mysterious jawbone and the Rolex are still missing after extensive further searches. No signs of a Sasquatch in the area either. The jawbone was last seen on the deceased and identified by five other persons. If it ever turns up, its holder will be a suspect in at least a theft and quite possibly a murder.

DUM DE DUM DUM, DUMMMM.

PART V – "A Monstrous Monstrosity"

The story continues. There'd been an accident during a rogaine and a man was found dead. Sgt. Joe NotFriday has urgent information for Chief Bruce Lawhead.

DUM DE DUM DUM, DUM DE DUM DUM, DUMMMM. *(Hum the theme now and then while you solve this.)*

A Tuesday, two months later, 8:30 AM. Captain Lawhead invited me into his office. He greeted me with a chuckle and said, "Well, Joe, bring me up to date on your Bigfoot monster case." I tried to ignore the animadversion. I told him I'd asked for this appointment because I'd awoken in a cold sweat at 2 AM night before last with an idea. The Chief interrupted to say that he often got his best "Aha's" that way. I'd called Ed Dowling, the police property room manager, and persuaded him to come with me to headquarters right then. We opened the evidence drawer. It was all there—the blood-stained rock, backpack with old patch, its contents just as the coroner had listed them, compass with lanyard, N*Swoosh envelope and memo, Toyota car key, red hat, hiking pole, sunglasses, and almost-new clothing and boots. No wristwatch was there, and no rings or other jewelry. The pack and the rock still held an evil smell. I looked carefully at each item, including everything in the pack, and puzzled over each one and how Knut was traveling very light. I checked the pants and boots—their size labels were missing; it looked like they'd been cut out I measured the boot length—12.5 inches, and the pant's length and waist. Later yesterday, I took the measurements to a department store here in Yakima. The boot length matched size 12, and the pants were the size for someone about 6'3" or 6'4", with a waist for someone likely to be over 200 pounds. Knut Phillips's driver's license showed: Height 6-04, Weight 215. Landchild advised that MacDonald, Ellsworth, and Waugh were also well over six feet tall.

I then went over key facts with the Chief, using my case notes (update attached). I pointed out the one key element Carl and I had missed earlier, and what it meant when supported by the rest of it and the new information I'd just reported. Captain Lawhead responded, "That's monstrous! Just think what went into all of this! This case is not what some of us of thought–a mishap or misadventure with a sasquatch. It's diabolical; it's a...a monstrous monstrosity!"

Seizing on this opening, I asked him to immediately call his contact in the FBI, and put a rush on the fingerprint results. He picked up the phone, called and received a quick answer that we can expect the report "any day now." I said with some disgust, "Right!"

After I went through the attached briefing notes encompassing the new developments in the case, the Chief ordered me not to wait but to get out an All Points Bulletin (APB) immediately. I asked, "What if I'm wrong?" He said, "My responsibility—do it, dammit!" I thanked him for his confidence in my reasoning, and went to find my partner Carl.

PHILLIPS'S CASE NOTES

Crime: Homicide? Suspicious death. Accidental (?) fall at Spiral Butte, White Pass, Hwy 12.

Coroner: Death due to massive head injury, instantaneous. Time of death estimated at 10 to 11 AM Sunday. No sign of foul play. Stomach ulcers present–not likely to be cause of fall. Body released for cremation.

Insurance Company: Investigation complete.

Conclusion: Accidental death due to fall. Investigator decided Sasquatch was a figment of imagination of tired and stressed people. Deputy Greenlee probably scared by natural rockfall from cliff. "No such thing as a Sasquatch!" Funeral go-ahead given.

Will: Dated one year ago. Witnessed. Everything to Kim. No other relatives. Cremation specified.

SUSPECTS (alphabetical):

Ellsworth: According to his former boss, Kent and he had a heated email dispute just after the death claim was filed over the size of insurance policy on Phillips. No discrepancies found in files or during investigation, and premiums were paid. Nevertheless, Kent resigned in a huff, apparently due to his integrity being questioned. Moved, left no forwarding address. Kim Stark not seen with him. Believed headed for Nepal in search of the Yeti.

Fulton: Confirmed that Phillips always wore a watch, and the Rolex he had was a new waterproof Oyster Perpetual. Told us that Phillips was top navigator, mountain climber, map reader, was right-handed, always wore glasses, and was in excellent physical shape, except for his stomach problem. He also said that Phillips had shaved off his moustache recently. See also "zag-zig" under ACTIVITIES. He confirmed rumors that he and Phillips would often get angry over some little incident, and throw things around, or at each other. But they'd never come to blows or injured each other or anyone else. Left last week for Yukon.

Hudson: With partner Peter Waugh won the next rogaine entered. N*Swoosh Company now sponsoring them, and they've begun a world promotional tour. Called twice to inquire how the investigation is going, and whether he can help. Thinks Phillips fell accidentally, because can't believe that any one person could have pushed or thrown Phillips off the cliff–unless very lucky. Now in Melbourne. Florida? Australia?

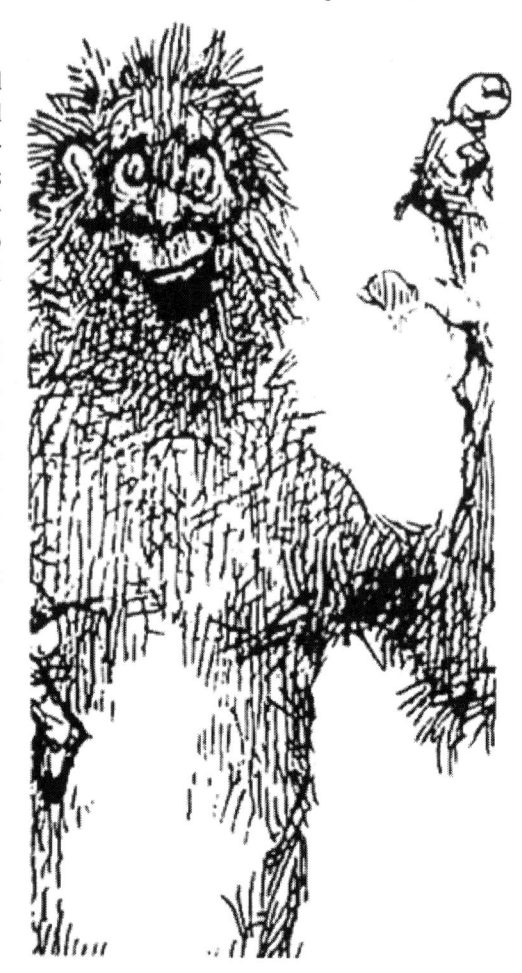

MacDonald: Seen leading twelve college students on lengthy field trips recently in the Spiral Butte area. His group spent a whole week near waterfall, according to Ardis Newell–Naches Ranger Station. Got into dispute with Ranger Susan Rykken on damage his group was doing to the wilderness environment there. Rykken said that MacDonald seemed obsessed with a quest for ancient artifacts, and they'd argued at length over ownership rights of any finds. Rykken also observed that Deputy Linda Jones was in his group, and was sharing a tent with him. Ranger Rykken commented on and seemed envious of Jones's blondness, youth, figure, and intelligence. MacDonald now reported on sabbatical leave, location unknown. Jones also on leave—coincidence?

Petty: Left word at his office that he was going off to unspecified locations for about two months on a "Bigfoot tracking expedition." Didn't say where. Has not been seen around the White Pass and Spiral Butte. Also left word that if the "cops" called, to tell them to go (✳□✈❄◆↓↘⇨🕒❄◆□!!!) themselves.

Sasquatch: (See insurance co. report) Carl's notes built plausible case for a Sasquatch retaliation–grabbing Knut up by the ankles, bouncing his face on a rock a few times, then dropping him over the cliff. Carl also has proposed an incredible solution involving a yetianthrope, or were-sasquatch (like a werewolf). Briefly: Phillips' "fatal" condition was increasingly frequent episodes of transformations into a sasquatch. His medication wore off under the stress of the rogaine at that last control. He had been trying to defeat other teams, then defect to the N*Swoosh camp for publicity,–but the unplanned episode occurred. Kim saw this, screamed, and others tried throwing rocks to scare off the now-Bigfoot. The animal ran around in fright and confusion, and accidentally fell off the cliff, hitting self with rock it grabbed to stop fall. Other rogainers watched as shape at foot of cliff returned to Phillips' form. The heptad agreed truth of accident would not be accepted, so conspired to tell various rock-throwing stories, but not mention the yetianthrope. Boomer detected the fearful sasquatch smell that Phillips could never get rid of completely. Kim and that jerk Petty later decided to be partly truthful, to protect themselves when we police started detailed questioning. Keg, the deputy who thought somebody was throwing rocks at him, by the way, is well known to have an overactive imagination. It was probably just a loose rock falling off of a cliff but he spooked and screamed himself before returning down Spiral Butte. Carl seems serious about all this. He and I disagree. Bigfoot location unknown.

Stark: Recently moved to Florida. Has post office box now in Miami. Apartment house neighbors said she moved with no friend's help. She seemed quiet and morose. No one's seen Ellsworth around her place recently, but they knew she had been living with him for a month or two before the accident. No street address in Miami.

Waugh: See Hudson. Also called to inquire on investigation. Offered only the trivia that he and Knut would often arm-wrestle after a rogaine; Waugh always lost, except sometimes won with his left arm. He and Hudson won easily in recent New Zealand rogaine. Tried weakly to convince me he and his partner did not do Phillips in. Now in Australia, according to Carol McNamara at N*Swoosh.

ACTIVITIES

Further searches in Spiral Butte area: No sign of jawbone, Rolex watch, other clues, nor Sasquatch signs. Rains have wiped out all footprints and ground disturbances.

Fulton told us on further questioning of the "zag-zig" technique he and Phillips used on several legs of the rogaine. Close on the heels of Team #3–their nemesis, Team #13 would see from the intention sheet that Peter and Fred were going, for example, for the left control of two about equally distant ahead. The next control after those was approachable equally well from either. So Fulton and Phillips would "zag" to the right control first, then head for the control that #3 was "zigzagging" to. They'd watch for the other team's route coming out of that control, but duck down and not reveal their own route as the other team passed. He remembered doing this about five times, and figured that they maybe gained ten to fifteen minutes overall on the other team. Several times they lost all contact with Team #3. Fulton argued that they never really broke the rule against deliberately following. Their routes just seemed to coincide. I asked who was making the final decision on his team when there was any difference of opinion on the best route. He said, "Phillips." I asked if they always split up for a one-to-five minute break after each control. He said, "Yes, we never changed that."

Phillips's friends contacted: Conversations with him in two months prior to mishap were that Knut was certain his stomach "cancer" would kill him soon. He gave each friend some memento from his possessions. Only five of them attended his funeral. Good thing he was cremated, or I would've had to help carry the casket. Neither Kim nor any other rogainers were there. Not a popular guy!

Kalon Stradeski contacted: Told us that the footprints he had seen in that loamy meadow with the tangled control bag were large shoe prints, not animal tracks. He didn't think an animal could have tangled up that bag the way it was.

Deputy Miller reported she and Boomer had been on several successful missing person searches recently, and Boomer is now ready to take her T.D.X. (advanced tracking) test. She still hasn't any idea why Boomer quit at Spiral Butte. Carl and I have a lead on that. We started with a phone call to (206) 625-POOP. Scatological, but fascinating!

END OF PHILLIPS'S CASE NOTES

1:00 AM. I told Carl about the briefing to the Chief and the APB (but not its contents), and that with any luck we'd have this case wrapped up shortly. He said, "Joe, that's fan-tas-tic, because the joke around the office is that you're the only one who doesn't think that Bigfoot did it. But, whooooodunit?"

I replied testily, "Carl, I think you're the one spreading that joke around. I'll show you the APB after I get it on the wire. You know, I only told the Chief about one of the ten clues we missed or paid no attention to. If we don't shape up, we might as well plan on going searching for your Sasquatch full time." I went down the hall to look up the words "monstrous" and "monstrosity" before writing the APB.

DUM DE DUM DUM, DUMMMM.

> "He did not stand shivering upon the brink, he was a thorough-paced liar, and plunged at once into the depths of your credulity."
> —Charles Lamb (1775-1834).

PART VI – Whodunit? "BIG-FOOT!"

The story concludes. There'd been an accident during a rogaine and a man was found dead. Sgt. Joe NotFriday has just finished briefing Chief Lawhead and telling his partner Carl Newson about the APB (all-points bulletin).

DUM DE DUM DUM, DUM DE DUM DUM, DUMMMM. *(Hum the theme now as you complete THE REAL DENOUEMENT.)*

11:30 AM. I finished sending off the APB to the world, and went looking for Carl, when Rick Landchild walked into our Yakima police precinct office. He had the final results report for the Spiral Butte Rogaine. I brought him up to date on the investigation, and reminded him of my deduction that Bigfoot killed "Big-Foot", or Knut Phillips. The insurance was paid out recently by registered mail to Kim Stark (Phillips' former girlfriend) at her P.O. Box in Miami, Florida. The insurance company had closed their investigation with an accidental death finding.

I surprised him with the news, "Now there's been another murder! Tell you about that in a few minutes. First, remember Carl Newson, my partner? He just went down the hall to pick up a fax. We got a lucky break. We did a local and FBI records check and fingerprint search on all the suspects. Chief Lawhead pulled a few political strings to move us up in the nine-month-long FBI work queue. The report's here now.

Let's see what you've got before he gets back."

Landchild reported, "Here's confirmation of that 'zig-zag' thing you called me about. (I corrected him: "zag-zig"). Fulton told you about that route scheme used by Team #13. The five controls Team #3 missed or had found concealed were the "zag" ones. While he was showing me the routes on the map, Carl walked in with the FBI fax. I showed Landchild the APB wire message the Chief had just released as Carl watched. Carl groused, "Oh, sure. Show him that first, then me. Some partner!" I retorted, "Can it, Carl. You're the guy fingering the Sasquatch. Read us what the FBI found." Carl read quickly, then summarized the report, "They've come up with something incredible!"

The fingerprints of Kent Ellsworth (he was Kim's partner/lover), taken at the campground parking lot that Sunday night of the rogaine, matched up with the prints for a known insurance fraud artist named Ken Burnett, from a case several years ago in Miami.

But get this: The prints of the deceased taken by the coroner in the morgue, supposedly the insured—Knut "Big-Foot" Phillips—matched the one on the bloody rock and hiking stick, as we knew. But they also matched the prints in US Army files from the Vietnam era for a Kent Ellsworth! Yes, Ellsworth." Carl said he'd suspected something like that all along. I said sarcastically, "Oh, suuuuure you did, Carl."

I'd suspected that a "Bigfoot" was the culprit. Now, reviewing the case, it all falls into place! It was all there:
—The deceased's TWO compasses (one even tied to his right wrist)—that Knut didn't use;
—The key to the wrong car (Toyota vs. Mazda) hidden under the gaiter;
—The glib use of the term "knackered" by "Ellsworth", a beginner rogainer;
—The extra time taken by Team #22 (Kim and "Kent") getting back;
—Knut's unbroken sunglasses, but with a smashed-in face on the corpse;
—'Kent's' facial first aid and foot treatment for non-existent sunburn and blisters—really a disguise applied by Kim;
—The phony (or was it?) bone; Kim's faked Sasquatch scream and sighting, and "Kent's" reporting of the scream;
—Les Petty matching the tracks he'd followed earlier with the boots on the Toyota and muddy tracks at the Hash House;
—Boomer alerting to Knut's continued presence in the parking lot after the body was taken away. Knut was right there in the Toyota as Deputy Miller and Boomer passed;
—Size 12 boots—but Knut had size 16 feet (I'd eventually woke up to check that!)

Boomer had worked it out, even after being put off by the planted scent from the backpack. Carl and I checked lots of places, and I found out that someone of Knut's description visited Woodland Park Zoo in Seattle and obtained some fresh tiger urine for "research" purposes. (An old tigress was having kidney problems.) I've recently learned that tracking dogs have phenomenal smelling powers not even half-way understood by humans.

All those clues! We should have solved it and had both of those clever murderers that Sunday night at Dog Lake! The car key was the real 'key,' to me. I'd keyed in on that one right away, but not the rest. The killers had missed it under the gaiter, and had stupidly missed the compass on the wrist.

"Big-Foot" was probably still worried about facial ID after dropping the body, so climbed down to make doubly sure of the job. Knut remembered his sunglasses then, and dropped them there. Another "sinister" aspect—it seems that Ellsworth was left-handed, and Phillips was right-handed. We had everyone's handwriting, and might have asked the coroner to determine handedness, but didn't. The compass was tied to the right wrist, for example—pointing to a lefty.

Knut probably never knew how close he came to getting knocked over that cliff himself, after planting all those false clues and getting rogainers angry at him. He and Kim must have timed their rendezvous to meet at Spiral Butte, hit Kent over the head, swap packs, and drop the body over the cliff. Kim knew her victim very well, living with him for two months. She had outfitted Kent with the same clothes and boots that Knut was wearing to the rogaine, so no one noticed any difference. With no face to look at, we all bought the rest of the ID. The phony jawbone (or was it a real find?) faked everyone out, as did the rock Knut fixed up. The foul smells in or on the pack and on the bogus N*Swoosh memo were put there to deter search dogs if called in. The smell was also planted to cast suspicion on the poor Sasquatch and support the accidental death finding. Knut, greedy at the last minute, couldn't bear to plant his expensive Rolex on the body but just took Kent's Casio watch off and wore it back, hiding his own.

I'm betting Kim Stark planned this whole diabolical thing. Just about everything she told us was a lie. She knew that her "lover" Kent had a bad case of stomach ulcers, which he'd told no one else about. She and Knut cleverly used that to help confirm the body identification. She probably had found the look-alike "fall guy" by chance right at the insurance office, bought the insurance from him, then set Ellsworth up for the kill!

Knut knew that Fulton liked to throw things when angry, and probably egged him on to throw a rock at him. Kim probably told MacDonald that she'd seen Fulton throw a rock and miss, but didn't want to tell the police and get him in trouble. I suspect she asked MacDonald, and maybe the others, to confirm that she'd seen one of them throw the rock and miss. All this to confuse the issue, leading to the many admissions of rock-throwing. Maybe they all did throw rocks. Makes no difference now.

Diabolical! I should have remembered the old detective saws about "Follow the money," and "Cherchez la femme."

Double indemnity—a cool $5 million. How sweet it must be! Kim and her "old flame" gained a lot for just seven months scheming! It almost worked cleanly, except for the disreputable anthropologist and the observant and crafty tracker. They almost caught the killers in the act! Knut also got back at that team of Peter and Fred for many past losses by tampering with control bags. They fooled us all!

Except Les Petty, the man-tracker. And Boomer, a dog that has deservedly earned her T. D. certification! Petty must have seen that his partner, MacDonald, was following the Phillips/Fulton team, and soon knew Knut's footprints. Then he saw Fulton's prints alone, crossing the marsh area going back to the HH finish. Back at camp, he noticed the size of the boots on Kent Ellsworth's car. Then—on the Hash House tent floor—he saw the fresh, muddy tracks of Knut, not Kent. Petty must have figured the scheme out right then, and saw how to profit by his knowledge. Too bad we ignored Boomer–we might have saved Les Petty. We traced Petty yesterday when we sought to confirm the above deductions. Unfortunately for Les, he was found dead last week with his head bashed in—in a vacant lot in Miami. A woman's big leather drawstring purse was nearby, covered in blood. Its only contents—a big brick! Miami police have no suspects. I know why he was down there—tracking down Kim and her boyfriend for a share of that $5 million by blackmail. So that's two murders—so far.

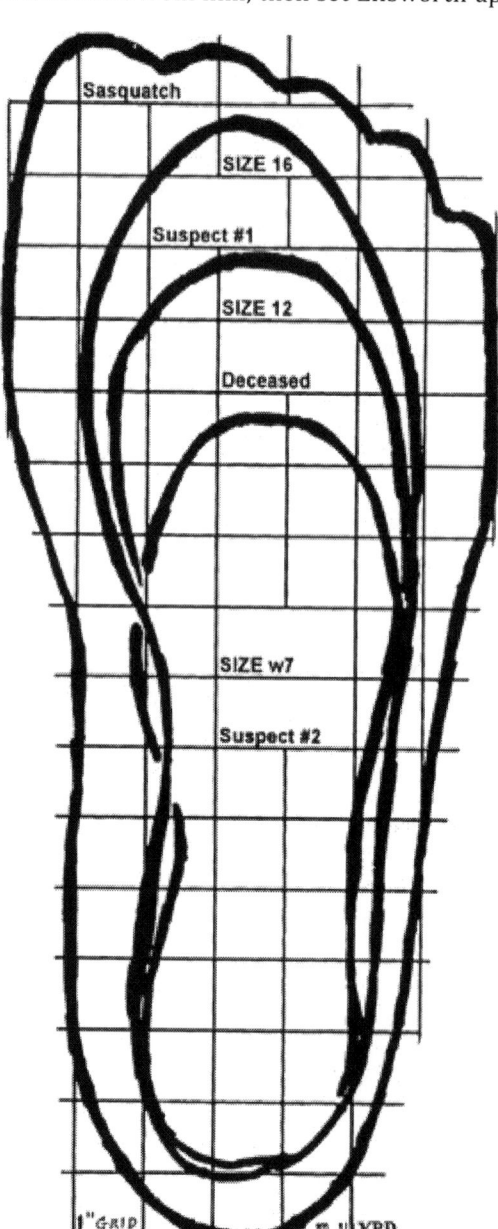

ONE WEEK LATER, 8:30 AM. Our APBs and INTERPOL queries to find Kim and Knut, or Kent, or Ken, or whoever "Big-Foot" is now, have given us no leads at all. I did call the Bellevue REI store, his usual outdoor gear source, who promised to help. I see there's going to be another rogaine—at Bald Mountain up near Spiral Butte—very soon. Carl says to pass the word, "Don't disturb the Sasquatch!" I think Carl needs a long vacation. As for me, I'll be heading on vacation to somewhere far away from con artists, mythical creatures, and murderers.

Carl and I have made mental notes to thank all those detectives who read our reports and assisted in solving this case. Yes, "Big-Foot" (size 16), not Bigfoot (an innocent and mythical bystander), really did kill "Big-Foot" (size 12).

10:20 AM. Ooops—the Bellevue REI store just called—vacation just canceled. I'm heading for Magnetic Island (a tropical paradise near Townsville, Queensland, Australia near the Great Barrier Reef) on business! Someone named Kurt Rowlands just sent in a mail order from there to the Lynnwood REI store (Ha! For once I anticipated Knut there!) for two custom pairs of size 16 hiking boots plus one pair of women's size 7 ($850 deposit!).

I've just gotten Chief Lawhead's approval for the trip after he asked why, since he'd heard that I was "apathetic" about the murders. I told him that Carl was wrong again; I'd said "ambivalent", meaning that I was astounded by the fiendishly clever plotting of the fraud, but disgusted with the viciousness of two suspects' malevolent murders. I've convinced the Chief that Kim and her partner are really living it up "down under". I'm taking the full-sized copy of the drawing (attached) that Margie York kiddingly drew up for my wall. And taking my scuba gear—just in case it's not them!

DUM DE DUM DUM, DUM DE DUM DUM, DUMMMM.

The story you've just read is not true. The names have been changed and scrambled to protect the innocent, who sometimes rogaine. Any resemblance to real persons or creatures living, mythical, or dead, is purely coincidental. For "Dragnet" fans, picture this story closing with A MARK II = VI PRODUCTION being hammered into stone. Coincidentally, Carl (who's also a mathematician) tells me if you move just one single element in the equation II = VI, it makes sense. Just like changing the one element of who actually died in the Spiral Butte case.

THE AUSTRALIAN PURSUIT – A Rogaining Misadventure

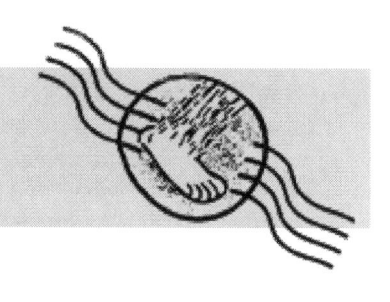

PART I – On the Trail of the Killers

It was early Sunday morning. 7:14 am. Foggy and overcast, with a threat of rain in Victoria in the Land of Oz. I was on an assignment Down Under, sent by the Sheriff's Office of Yakima County, Washington State, the USA. Pursuing two murderers. My name's NotFriday. I carry a badge, number 714. I'm a cop.

DUM DE DUM DUM, DUM DE DUM DUM, DUMMMM. *(The reader is encouraged to hum the Dragnet theme music now and then throughout this story.)*

At 9:42 AM, Detective Sergeant Gordy Holman from the Victoria State Police picked me up for the drive to the 6-hour metrogaine in Bendigo, northwest of Melbourne. His oversized LandCruiser, otherwise unmarked as official, was fitted out with a big 'roo' bar on the front, police radios, and even a GPS receiver. I asked about how often he had encountered kangaroos on the highways around Victoria. "Seldom happens," he said, "and I've never hit one, but I've seen maybe a dozen vehicles that have. Those without these bars suffered about as much damage as the 'roos."

I mentioned that I'd nearly hit a deer driving from Yakima to Seattle on this trip. He asked if my trip otherwise was OK. I frowned and said, "Well, not exactly. First, there was the security checker who was found asleep at his station at Sea-Tac. Caused a shutdown of most of the airport for hours while they rechecked all the passengers, including those on my flight, which was ready to taxi and was recalled to the gate. Then there was the missing wallet snafu in San Francisco, when my wallet went through the scanning belt and fell off the end into some space under the security station. That took 20 minutes to retrieve.

'Then my credit card got stuck in the automatic teller machine at Sydney airport. I was trying to find out where to report it, when a woman walked up, tried her card, and the machine spat mine back out. I thought that was about enough for one trip, but at the Melbourne Airport my luggage got checked by the sniffer dog, and that beagle found a very interesting smell. His handler had to hand-search all my bags. The beagle meanwhile focused on the food pouch on the handler's belt, awaiting a handout for the job. I never learned what the smell was, but it could have been a banana skin or a partly-eaten Clif Bar I had forgotten about after an orienteering event.

"But all those happenings paled to insignificance when compared to stuff in the Horwitz book I was reading on the plane about Capt. James Cook's voyages back in the 1770s. He took almost two years to do the trip I was not comfortable making in about 20 hours, and he lost over 40% of his crew in doing so to punishments, bad diet, accidents, venereal diseases and desertions."

Gordy Holman commented, "Well, then you read about Cook's ghastly end. Your Hawaiian natives were more attuned to what Cook was up to than our Aborigines. They deboned him!"

I replied, "Yeah, so we gained a 50th state eventually; meanwhile you guys still honor the Queen.

"But one good and memorable thing happened—I saw a 'glory' as we circled to land at Melbourne. Know what that is?"

Detective Holman (he said to call him Gordy) said, "Never heard of it."

I rambled on, "It's similar to the Specter of Brocken—which mountain-climbers sometimes see at sunrise. The sun, directly behind or above you, casts a giant shadow of you, or the airplane you're in, on a cloud or fog bank. The sun's rays are reflected back to you like a rainbow, with multicolor bands. But in the case of a 'glory', you see a complete circle around the shadow of your airplane. I asked our pilot about

Published in *Orienteering North America* April through October 2003 issues.

it after we landed. He said pilots see them often, but his technical explanation didn't sound quite right. I'll have to check it when I get back home with Don, my weather expert in Seattle.

"You know, that incident with the beagle reminded me of the clue we missed during the murder investigation of that rogaine event back in 1994—this case that I'm still on now."

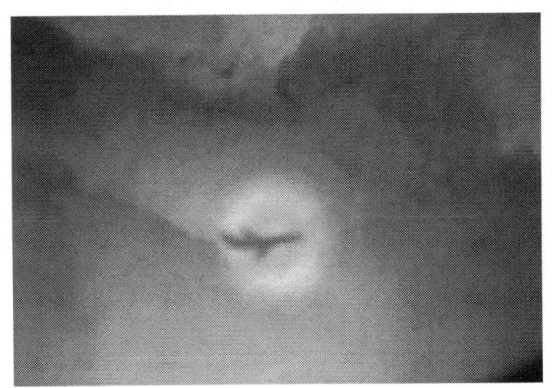

"Yeah, tell me about that. I heard that you figured out the murder just a little too late," Gordy interjected.

"It was a little embarrassing, but my partner Carl and I were somewhat distracted by some red herrings and too many suspects, including a possible sasquatch. I hear you call red herrings 'furphies', but..."

Gordy interrupted, "A sasquatch—what's that?"

"You may have heard of it as a Bigfoot, the perhaps mythical creature, a big, seven to eight foot primate, nocturnal, that's been reported for centuries in almost every state in the USA and in many countries worldwide. No one's ever killed one, or found a body that we know of, but many finely detailed footprints have been found, showing even broken bones and sweat glands, plus hair and other signs that can't be explained."

In the case of a "glory," you see a complete circle around the shadow of your airplane

"Oh yeah, we've got the Yowie reports here in Australia, mostly in the mountainous areas in the east, but a few reports also from here in western Victoria. Vicious creature per reports—attacks man and beast when provoked, or sometimes just when hungry. Never been caught here, either. Most people think it's just folklore or people having fun or playing tricks. But I can't imagine anyone crazy enough to dress up in an ape costume and run around at night. Just about guaranteed to be blown away by the first rancher or farmer who got a chance for a shot.

"We also get reports of big feral cats, like panthers in size, stalking sheep and cattle around here. No native animals like that known here in Oz. Of course we've got a wild collection of unique flora and fauna, like 12-foot worms. Plus crop circles! Hope you get a chance to see some while you're here. Go on, mate, tell me more about your case."

> "As a rule, the more bizarre a thing is, the less mysterious it proves to be."
> — Sherlock Holmes

"The murder took place during a rogaine at White Pass, Washington back in 1994. That's a mountainous area between Yakima and Mt. Rainier in the Cascade Mountain Range. A rogainer, first identified as Knut Phillips, fell to his death off Spiral Butte, an old volcanic cone near the campground at Dog Lake. We investigated, questioned the many witnesses among the other rogainers, had a search dog team on hand, and collected a jawbone, a bloody rock and other items connected with the death. We concluded that we couldn't be sure that it was other than an accident or maybe an angry sasquatch encounter, so we released all the witnesses that night That was my blunder.

"It wasn't long, though, before some of the clues started to make sense. For example, the deceased was left-handed, but we learned later that Knut Phillips was right-handed. The dead man also carried compasses that Knut would never have used—he was a thumb-compass man. Then there was the car key tied to the deceased's boot, which did not fit Knut's car. A Rolex watch Knut was seen wearing was missing. And then there were the statements made by Kim Stark and her boyfriend "Kent." This turned out to be a well-done charade. I have to admit, though, I had help in solving this case. Les, rogainer at the event, spotted big footprints and matched them to the murderer, who was masquerading as Kent."

"You're saying that Kim and Kent killed a mate named Knut, switched identities, and made it look like an accident. Looks like they planned it well."

"Actually, Kim and Knut killed Kent, making it look like it was Knut who died. It was a big-payoff double-indemnity insurance scam. What really burned me was when my superiors ignored what the tracker dog Boomer tried to tell us, when she sniffed out the missing (supposedly dead) man in the parking lot, long after the deceased's body had been taken away. It wasn't until I checked the boot size of Kent, the real deceased, that I had enough to convince my boss what had happened. That sniffer beagle at your airport reminded me of Boomer.

"We put out an all-points bulletin, never found either Knut or Kim, but later learned that Les, the gumshoe/rogainer, had followed them to Miami Florida to capture them and collect the reward money. But Les was killed by a blow to the head much like the one that had killed Kent at Spiral Butte. So I'm after two double-murderers. And I'm carrying warrants for their arrest."

"Looks like a tough job, and I remember you told me you have no photos, no fingerprints, no DNA. and only shoe sizes and rough descriptions to go on. So you think maybe you'll actually corner them here?"

"Well, as I mentioned in my fax to you, they were last traced to Magnetic Island near Townsville, Queensland back in 1995. Knut, using his real name for some dumb reason, ordered some custom-made boots for himself and Kim. Sizes 16 and 7. The two "big-foots" I'm after.

'Then they left a forwarding address to a post office box in Melbourne, which I found had been closed out. Another dead end. Then, just last week, I got a call from the local cops in Bendigo. Michelle Matthews, an orienteering meet director who was hanging posters for an upcoming event saw the wanted poster of Knut and Kim. She said she had seen two rogainers who matched the general description of those two. She alerted us that they were entered in this Bendigo Metrogaine. She gave us their names, and also reported they were registered for the big 24-hour rogaine starting next weekend at Enfield."

Gordy thought for a minute, while driving furiously on what was to me the wrong side of the road! He said, "You know, I can arrest them, but we're going to need rock-solid proof that we've got the right mongrels."

"You're right, Gordy, and we'll need enough to convince one of your judges for an extradition. Do you think we will get to this metrogaine before the noon start?"

Gordy checked the odometer and his watch and said, "No worries, mate, she'll be apples. This Bendigo Metrogaine will start from the city park and ballfield right in town. We should have some time to wander around ourselves, and not tip off the suspects of what we're about. I see you've brought your backpack. What all have you got in your kit?"

I thought about my packing job. "Well, pretty much the stuff the rogainers back in Washington recommended: some extra clothes (in my case a set of synthetic underwear and a lightweight rain suit, a balaclava face mask, and light gloves) a small knife, lighter, fire-starting block of wood fiber and a candle, sunglasses, my pills, tiny first aid kit, a world-wide balanced compass and a spare, a small flashlight, sunglasses, a headlamp, a space blanket, several Clif Bars, a Camelbak water bladder, some moleskin and blister ointment, and a 50 foot line of parachute cord. Oh, also a pencil and notebook for work. And I tried hard to keep it down to 10 pounds, like those rogainers back home recommended."

Gordy seemed astounded. "Goodonyer! Looks like you're equipped for a 24-hour classic. Did you remember to bring a whistle?"

"Yeah," I answered, "and I wear it around my neck. Heard of people who, when they needed help quickly, couldn't find or reach their whistle. So I keep it real handy. Oh, I also brought a little magnetic chess set, because I heard a rumor that you play chess. If we get time for a break somewhere, maybe we'll get in a game. This metrogaine – is it like those they're just starting up in the States this year? Mostly run on city streets and parks, with the teams trying to get to as many features as possible in the time allotted?"

"Right, mate," Gordy replied as he drove even faster. "Rogaine clubs have been doing these metrogaines for many years in this country. Lots of people enjoy them, since it gets them out to new towns and cities they often haven't visited before, and it's almost like a guided tour of the highlights and historical points of the place. Still requires careful navigation and route planning, with too many places, or controls, to get to before the time runs out. Beginners and less-skilled navigators like these city events, which don't pose the off-trail and climbing dangers and night navigation challenges that the 24-hour bush events do."

I asked how he knew all that. He chuckled and said his wife rogaines a lot, but he quit years ago after acquiring a 'crook' knee.

We arrived at the Bendigo downtown city park, and checked in with the organizers at their tent on the ball field. Their welcome sign had a sample map and aerial photo of the area, and highlighted that their Victorian Rogaining Association had been running 24-hour rogaines since 1947, and metrogaines since 1985. Michelle "Shelly" Matthews, the meet director who had notified the authorities, took us off to a quiet spot and introduced herself.

"G'day, mates. I'm Shelly, and we're glad to see you here. I understand no one is to know who you are – you're just beginner rogainers, here to give this a go. But I've got bad news. It seems that those two I told you about, Kurt Taylor and Kath Smith, have cancelled out. That's according to Kurt's business partner, who arrived a short time ago. But he said they'd be at the rogaine this next weekend at Enfield."

"Too bad. Maybe we can ask his partner a few things, but don't let him know who we are either. What do you know about him?"

"His name is Michael Aylott, and that's about all I know about him. Since the meet is about to start, you can probably catch him at the finish at 6 PM. We'll have lots of food after the rogaine, and I think he said he wants to distribute a bunch of flyers on the investment venture he and Kurt are promoting. I'm sure both those blokes are iilywhackers. Here's one he gave me."

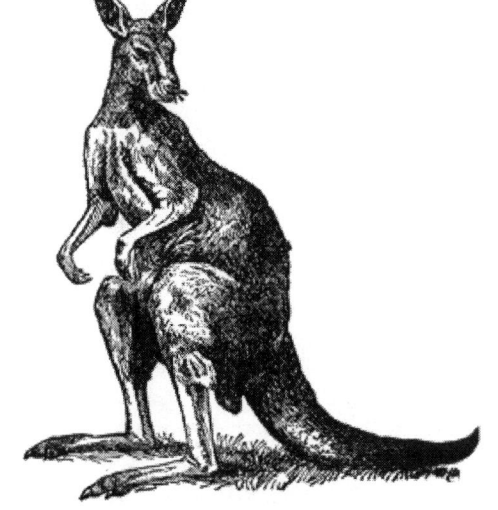

I looked at the flyer. It was a fancy color brochure outlining a business venture which involves the building of a new, giant gold-ore-dredging ship in the Yukon up in Canada. The photo showed a huge, stern-wheeler river boat, like those used 100 years ago near Whitehorse. The pamphlet talked about finding lots of low-grade gold ore in the Yukon River, and the studies showing the feasibility of re-dredging the river for the remainders left of the dredging done back in the 1906-1920 era. It listed the contact point for obtaining a prospectus for investing in stock in the corporation formed to develop this enterprise, build the ship, mine the river, and sell the gold.

I asked Shelly for a description of our two suspects. She said that Kurt Taylor was rather tall, over six feet, had a scruffy beard, those large feet she'd noticed, and had a 'Yankee' accent. His sheila, Kath Smith, was short, peroxided, big-muscled, and some facial plastic surgery noted recently by other rogainers. She draws the pervish glances of all the blokes the way she walks and dresses. She also had large feet for her height.

"Since you two are at loose ends until 6," suggested Shelly, "how about entering this metrogaine. You'll get to see the interesting things around Bendigo, including the Loong and Sun Loong Chinese dragons, a Chinese Garden, the old Deborah mine, a train museum, art gallery, a Joss House, and some reminders of the bushrangers who used to rob the gold shipments out of here. Kind of a self-guided tour of the town, which has a population of about 90,000 now."

Following a brief discussion, with many reassurances from Shelly, we decided to do the event. She warned us that some signs of a yowie had been reported in the bush near the city. Mainly torn out road signs with their posts impossibly twisted (not snapped) in two. And some faint footprints.

Gordy laughed and told us that the yowie probably exists only in the imaginations of some alkies and drongos. And grinning, he said that, anyway, they only come out at night, like vampires.

We quickly looked over the course, picked a few close-in controls, including some with high pointers, and started off with the mass start 'quest' (as Shelly called them) of rogainers. We looked more like a mob of kangaroos, scattering in all directions just as the Sun finally broke through the overcast. I told Gordy that the meet director back at Spiral Butte had explained how they set these courses so that the point values are balanced around the venue. He looked, did some addition in his head, and confirmed that there were no high-pointed groupings, and any half of the map almost exactly matched the other half in control point totals.

On one early leg to a control, I checked my map to confirm that our route was approximately due west at that point, and then started to look at my new, world-balanced compass. But my own shadow caught my eye – it was there to the left of me. I immediately got an unsettled, disoriented feeling. My shadow told me I had to be going east, not west! My compass said otherwise. Then, the image of a wallaby seen just an hour ago flashed through my mind's eye. With a jolt, I realized the sun was now in the north at noon, not south! I mused, "We're not in Kansas anymore, Toto!"

After two hours of collecting control points, we stopped for lunch at a small deli near a control at a park. The sun had warmed the air, so we moved to an outdoor table. The peg-board chess set came out of my backpack. In the first game, Gordy caught me with the hoary old Legal's Mate, with the game over in a few moves after I grabbed his poisoned Queen. Starting a second game, Gordy drew my attention to a rogaine team walking by, studying their maps. He whistled under his breath and commented on the short, good-looking, dark-haired girl. The two rogainers vanished down a side street, and we laughed when they soon reappeared, rechecked their maps, and starting running down the block in the opposite direction.

Gordy chuckled, "You know, mate, humans are the only creatures who, when they lose their way, run faster!"

Maybe this distraction helped because I quickly crushed him with a Queen sacrifice. Disgusted, Gordy threw the board across the park into a bush. Then, laughing, he ran to retrieve it and returned it to my backpack. We resumed our metrogaine wanderings.

As we were passing by a candy store, Gordy pushed me in and said he had to get me something. He bought three small figures wrapped in foil, and handed them to me. They were chocolate figures of Yowies, made by Cadbury. I laughed and said when we see a pharmacy I'd get him a gift, too – some Rogaine, since it looked like he was starting to need it.

We nailed a few more controls and then jogged a bit to get back to the finish before 6 PM, knowing that we'd lose 10 points a minute for being late.

Gordy and I finished up at the Hash House, the outdoor patio of a restaurant right in town. We went over what our approach would be during our chat with the suspect's business partner Mike Aylott. His team arrived back just about 6, and sat down to eat. We joined them, looking like just another knackered rogaine team, which we actually were! His partner turned out to be the good-looking gal that Gordy had seen earlier. He introduced her as his secretary, Jane Clarke. She told us this was her first rogaine. With the gold dredging pamphlet in hand, we feigned interest in the investment, while getting what we could on his partner.

I commented on his fancy Rolex watch, saying how I'd been shopping for a used one on eBay recently, with the same three small dials. He said his partner Kurt had given it to him, because Kurt's girlfriend Kath had bought him a newer, even more ostentatious one. I said it looked great, showing little signs of wear and a new one like that goes for over $10,000 US dollars. Aylott said that he was surprised that it didn't have a scratch on it, for he knew that Kurt wore it everywhere, including on many rogaines he said he'd done. I smiled and nudged Gordy under the table. But Gordy was focusing on Jane's departing figure, as she excused herself and went to their car to bring back a six-pack of Fosters.

DUM DE DUM DUM, DUM DE DUM DUM, DUMMMM.

PART II–The Cassowary, the Dredge, and the Letter

Following the Bendigo Metrogaine, my partner Gordy Holman of the Victorian State Police and I were completing our questioning of Michael Aylott, the business partner of Knut Phillips a.k.a. Kurt Taylor, our suspected murderer. I was on an assignment Downunder, sent by the Sheriff's Office of Yakima County, Washington State, the USA. Pursuing two murderers. My name's NotFriday. I carry a badge, number 714. I'm a cop.

DUM DE DUM DUM, DUM DE DUM DUM, DUMMMM. *(The reader is encourage to hum the Dragnet theme music now and then throughout this story.)*

Sunday, 6:30 PM: I made up a story that I was looking into insurance now for my own company, and asked Aylott about the details. He told us he and Kurt Taylor started the corporation two years ago. Started gathering data, plans, and began promoting to investors. Preliminary trips to Yukon Territory in Canada. Set up accounting, insurance, and brokerage network. Got key-man life insurance on partners. He said that the AU $10 million policies cost AU $100,000 each. He had concluded that was not too bad, and a write-off that the investors were covering.

"I understand your partner has done several rogaines. Have you done these often?"

"No, this is my first, and I'll be trying the 24-hour one this weekend. My associate Kurt Taylor is also competing, but with his girlfriend Kath Smith. I'll be running with Ben Baldwin, who's done these before. But Ben has a 'crook' knee, so we won't be moving very fast, but it still should be fun."

"Have a picture of your partner? I may have rogained with him in Queensland some years back."

"I've got a poor little picky here in my wallet I took a few months back of Kurt and Kath at an outing we took to see the penguins at Phillip Island. Take a look." (He laughed). "They were chasing two little penguins, and I caught them in the act. They don't ever like their pictures taken, so I keep this out of their sight."

I didn't recognize Kurt, but maybe it's that heavy beard. And Kath looked nothing like the gal I remembered from that murderous rogaine in Washington. Aylott told me that Kurt is an American who moved here many years ago. Kurt's partner, Kath Smith, is somewhat younger, short, platinum blonde, very flashy, with long nails, expensive jewelry, and with enough silicon added to make her unsinkable. He told me that in just the past two years she's had two plastic surgeries on her nose and face, and has gone from a dark blonde to a silver peroxide, not to mention a bust enhancement that is phenomenal.

"She's quite a knockout in such a short package. And she's been seen lifting heavy weights in workouts."

I got his business card and another copy of his brochure, and promised to look into the opportunity further.

The awards were given out then, going to teams in various categories. They used self-scoring control cards that speeded up the preparation of results. Seemed that all teams received something, and half the teams got a place award, but they were all inexpensive, handcrafted mementos. I wondered why people did this sport, with no big sponsors, no spectators, no TV coverage, no newspaper reporters, only token prizes, and plenty of blisters. Everyone looked tired but happy. I didn't bother to ask them why they rogained.

We helped the organizers by picking up two of the control markers on our way out of the area. Shelly, the meet director, told us that she'd learned long ago that many rogainers, even after a tough competition, were willing to help clean up the Hash House area and retrieve controls. I remembered that back in Washington they called this the "one control pickup."

I thought it was unlikely to be just a coincidence that my two murderers would pursue the same obscure sport here that they had used to cover a capital crime in the States. Except for their heights, though, there was not much else to go on, except shoe sizes. I looked over my checklist, which was very short:

Male (Knut Phillips):
- Over six feet tall
- Caucasian

- Est. age 40-50
- Beard, mustache, or clean-shaven
- Shoe size 16
- Right handed
- Wears Rolex watch always
- Competes in rogaines
- Rarely uses a compass
- Was in Queensland, Australia in 1995 (known because of REI boot order)
- Last known address in Melbourne, Australia

Female (Kim Stark):
- Under five feet tall
- Caucasian
- Blonde (natural?)
- Muscular
- Est. age 35 – 45
- Shoe size W7
- Talkative
- Competes in rogaines
- Suspected to use bludgeon or rock on a rope
- Last known address in Melbourne, Australia

Thursday, 11 AM: Detective Holman took me to downtown Melbourne to the corporate offices of the gold dredge investment venture pair: Kurt Taylor and his partner Michael Aylott. Just before entering the fancy address, I paused to look over a dark blue Toyota Prius dual gas-electric car, parked at the curb nearby. Looked like an ideal vehicle for urban commuting, with gas prices probably going up every year. Gordy led me into the office. Only Jane Clarke, the young secretary we'd met at the metrogaine, was in. She looked even better in the office lighting, with her long dark hair, amazing figure, and cute face all on a five-foot frame. She said that Mr. Taylor and Mr. Aylott were both traveling, one to Sydney and one to Launceston. Told us they wouldn't be back until late Friday. No pictures of them were available. But she said both planned to enter the Enfield Rogaine on Saturday. She invited us to look at the displays in their big conference room. I wandered around, but Gordy was more interested in sitting down at her desk and conversing.

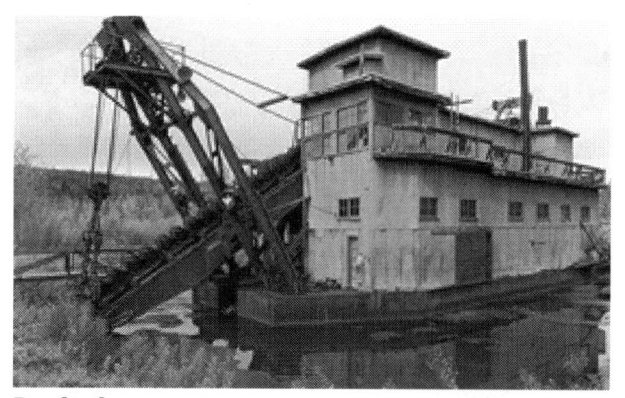

Dredge boat.

A large stuffed cassowary was on a lighted display stand at one end of the room. Looked about 4 feet tall, 130 pounds, with bluish armor plate on its head. Flightless bird with deadly claws on its feet. Sign said, 'Taken by Kurt Taylor, Queensland, 1995.' I took a picture.

I wandered around some more, first looking at a big scale model of a dredge boat named "Alice May" in a riverbed in a large glass-covered display in their conference room. The model detail was obviously the work of professional model-makers, and very expensive. Parts all labeled. The walls held pictures and news articles from various places where gold was mined in the past century.

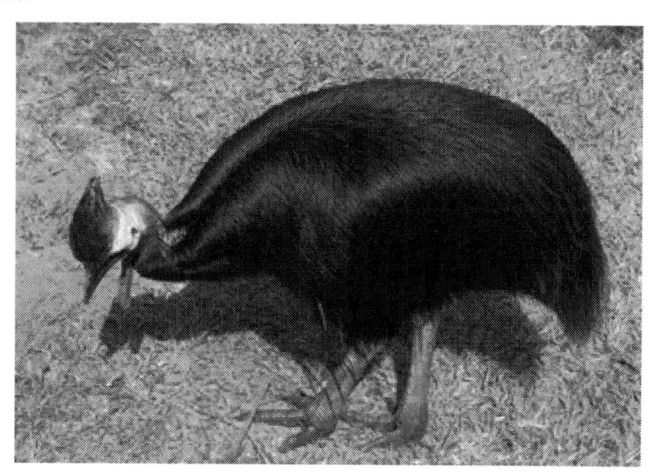

There was a framed letter from the mayor of Whitehorse, Yukon Territory, welcoming the company and cheering their plans to re-dredge the Yukon River nearby. Something caught my eye—a single spelling error. Then another clue—a small defect in the leg of the letter "y" everywhere in the text.

Hanging next to the letter was a poem "The Cremation of Sam McGee" by Robert W. Service. And a framed laboratory certificate reporting the favorable results of a sample dig from the Yukon River.

Another wall held a large artistic print of an ape-like creature emerging from the forest. It was labeled "A Yowie in Victoria?"

I re-examined the labels on the dredge parts, read a line of the poem, and then snapped a few close-ups with my digital camera.

Spotting the copying from Robert Service, I thought about how everything I'd seen here had the earmarks of a confidence man who just dared people to catch him in his rotten schemes. I felt sure psychiatrists had a name for this—made note to look it up.

Back in the main office, I found my partner Gordy still in deep conversation with Jane Clarke. A few cheap-looking rogaining awards and maps were displayed on a shelf. Dated from 1995 to earlier this year. Besides the newest model computer, a large wall-mounted plasma-screen TV, and fancy fax and dictating equipment, I noticed an old IBM Selectric typewriter on a typing desk in the corner. Curious, I looked closely at it. I asked Ms. Clarke if it was OK to try it, since it looked like the kind my mother had back in the '70s. She nodded OK, and I inserted a sheet and typed "the sly quick brown fox jumped over the lazy, lazy dog." Stuffing the sheet in my pocket, I commented on how "cool" that old machine was, and how sad it was that all the other sophisticated gear had made such equipment obsolete. She just nodded again, and I signaled to Gordy that we should go. He thanked Jane for her information on the company, while slowly shaking her hand much too long.

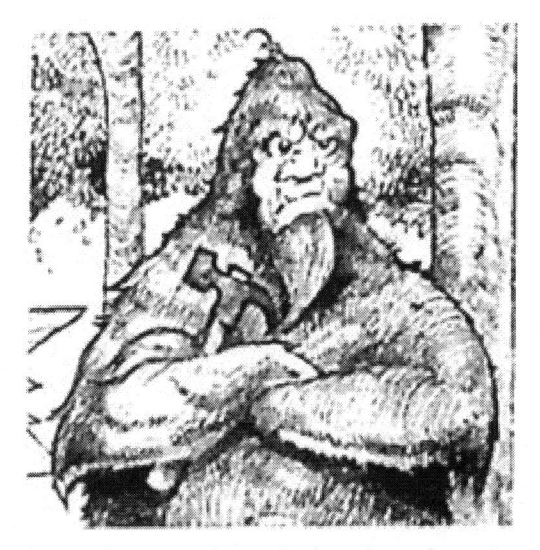

We walked down the block and stopped for lunch. Gordy covered quickly what he had learned. Jane had blabbed on and on that both her bosses were raking in lots of investment money spending it like crazy on car leases, the fancy office, expensive key-man insurance, several trips to Canada, ship models, plans and artwork, and a nice salary for her. They'd also rented a hunting cabin up around Kerang for a week, and were having her bring some gear up there this weekend for after the rogaine.

"She said those two had been spending all their spare time, along with Kath Smith, searching for a live yowie. She's going to be carrying their big-bore rifles, ammo, night vision goggles, radios, GPSs, and lots of food and Foster's up there. She said that in her opinion they're all crazy." I thought she's the one who's crazy here, working for these nefarious people who'd get rid of her in an instant if they knew how much she was revealing about their operations.

I told Gordy about the stuffed cassowary bird and the Yowie print. He said the cassowary was a protected species, even back in 1995. He was irate at the idea of one being shot and openly displayed today.

Concerning the yowie, he told me that he'd never believed reports of the creature. But just three years ago some ranger near Sydney came across a grove of prehistoric trees called Nightcap Oak that scientists were sure went extinct more than 10,000 years ago. So he's never very surprised when things like 12-foot worms and panthers turn up for real in Oz. In addition, he said 'Taswegians' are still reporting spotting the extinct Tasmanian Tiger, gone since 1936.

I responded that the first person that captures or kills a yowie, sasquatch, yeti, or whatever will be world famous, and the second person to do so will undoubtedly go to jail.

Gordy added, "Oh, heh, heh, by the way, she asked if I might meet her for a Foster's at a pub here when she gets back. I asked if they just shut the office down while they're all gone. She said their answering machine picks up all their calls, and they use cell phones and laptops to get their messages."

I showed Gordy the paper I'd typed on the Selectric. Told him to examine the tails of the "y's" in the text. He spotted the little defect. I told him all the labels on the dredge display had the same defect. I noted how interesting it was that the framed letter from the Whitehorse mayor I'd just seen had the same font and the same "y" defect in it. So did the lab report on the placer gold dig samples.

He grinned and observed, "Looks like Shelly was right about this operation being a big scam."

On leaving the restaurant, we waited for a tram to pass, and then started to go to our truck across the street. But I forgot the left-hand driving here for a moment, looking left, not right as we stepped out. Gordy jerked me back as a blue Toyota just brushed. Gordy pointed out that we were jaywalking, so wouldn't have had much of a defense if we'd been hit. He reported that he got a glance at the driver, who didn't pause, and said it shocked him that it was she—Jane Clarke. I wondered if she deliberately tried to hit us. I commented that the car was so quiet I didn't even hear it coming.

> "Somewhere, something incredible is waiting to be known."
>
> — Carl Sagan

Thursday, 3 PM: We returned to Detective Holman's office, and prepared for our trip Saturday to the Enfield-Jubilee Rogaine. Web pages gave us sunrise and sunset times, moon phase, magnetic declination, and the weather forecast. Weather report predicted overcast, possible showers, after heavy rainfall Friday. Gordy noted we would not see much of the moon Saturday night, even though planners scheduled major rogaines for full moons. I rechecked my backpack, making sure I had my Gore-Tex coat and Seattle sombrero, rainproof pants, and fresh batteries plus spares for my headlamp and small flashlight. Also a second whistle as a zipper-pull on my coat. Didn't feel good about not having my handgun, but decided Gordy's Glock should be sufficient. He told me he had a spare hidden in his truck.

Holman checked with the experts on extradition procedures—our identification information so far looked shaky. We chewed over the possibilities of how to prove that Taylor and Smith were my murderers.

DUM DE DUM DUM, DUM DE DUM DUM, DUMMMM.

PART III – Death at the Enfield-Jubilee Rogaine

Following the Bendigo Metrogaine, my partner Gordy Holman of the Victorian State Police and I had questioned Michael Aylott, the business partner of Knut Phillips a.k.a. Kurt Taylor, our suspected murderer. We had visited their office and talked with their secretary Jane Clarke, and were now on our way to the 24-hour rogaine west of Melbourne. I was on an assignment Down Under, sent by the Sheriff's Office of Yakima County, Washington State, the USA. Pursuing two murderers. My name's NotFriday. I carry a badge, number 714. I'm a cop.

DUM DE DUM DUM, DUM DE DUM DUM, DUMMMM. *(The reader is encouraged to hum the Dragnet theme music now and then throughout this story.)*

Saturday, 8 AM: Gordy was hunched over the wheel driving his LandCruiser like a lunatic again, heading west on CityLink, then out of Melbourne. Nearing Ballarat, he said, "Well, I thought we'd have plenty of time, but look ahead. Some big traffic pileup up there. I'll check on my police band and see what's up." We heard radio traffic, much channel switching, and then a traffic report.

"Looks bad, mate—we talked about kangaroo strikes—seems we have one up ahead, with injuries to the driver and passengers. There'll be a delay while they get the St. John ambulance in and clear the highway. Looking at this map, we may as well wait it out, since it's a long backtrack to take the southern route in. What's worse, there are reports of local flooding of some bush roads and a few main routes due to heavy rains. We're in the midst of a 100-year drought, with sheep dying by the tens of thousands and wells drying up, but we still get these bloody spot storms. We've even had tourist groups on camels trapped in the outback when surrounded by flash flooding."

I mentioned to Gordy something that disturbed me about the model of the gold dredge at the investment office we'd visited Thursday. The dredge had a huge paddlewheel for propulsion, but it seemed that the photos and articles posted there had the old dredges just pulling themselves slowly along the bottom with their scoop shovels. Didn't make sense to me. Gordy remarked, "Mate, maybe sternwheeler steamboats are coming back. Big deal I hear now for gambling on your Mississippi River. Which reminds me, did you know that your Mark Twain spoke here in Melbourne about his piloting experiences?"

I asked, "When was that?" He told me it was a famous speech at the Yorick Club in 1895. He also said facetiously that if anyone really wanted to invest in that gold dredge, he had a real sweet deal for him or her in a coalmine in Wonthaggi.

Just then, a big kangaroo came bounding across the road ahead of us, moving at an amazing speed. She had a joey in her pouch, enjoying the ride. Just more bigfeet in this case.

Gordy then told me of some research he'd done yesterday, after seeing a possible pattern or m.o. of our suspects. He'd checked old case files on murders and accidents around Magnetic Island in Queensland since 1995. One closed case involved the apparent drowning of a man off a cruise boat on a tour of the Great Barrier Reef in 1997. Parts of his shark-eaten body were found. A business partner, who was not in the state at the time, heavily insured the man. But that partner, named Kirk, had a girlfriend who was on the same boat with the deceased when he disappeared. I asked the girlfriend's name. He said, "It was Kyla Stone."

I observed that they both must have monogrammed handkerchiefs! I told Gordy of my dinner engagement Friday night. A gold mining expert, Neil Plunkett-Cole from the local University and I went to a late dinner, after attending his nephew's cello concert. I showed him the brochure from the dredge venture, and he estimated it would take about 100 years to get a payback on the deal as proposed.

Gordy responded, "No surprises there, mate. I knew those drongos were running a con. What did he play?"

"Play? What? Oh, you mean the nephew. It was Solo Cello Suite No. 1 by Derek Strahan, an Aussie. He sounded like another Yo-Yo Ma developing. Oh, and I got a parking ticket for being in a restricted neighborhood zone at night. Maybe you can fix it for me?"

Gordy laughed, and asked me to pass the ticket and a pen. Driving one-handed, he scrawled something on it, signed it with a flourish, and passed it back. I gave out an exaggerated groan when I read, "OK to pay." Laughing, Gordy finally gave up on the creeping traffic, put a flashing light on his roof, and drove the shoulder to bypass the backup.

Saturday, 12:15 PM: We finally arrived at the event center, called the Hash House, a few minutes too late for the mass start. We passed a few teams running down the road as we drove in. I pounded the dashboard and cursed our luck at having missed seeing our suspects once again. I had to talk to them and see if they were the ones.

We met the head "Organiser," Geoff Costigan, explained our mission, and urged secrecy. He told us that the "quest" of rogainers were off after points on a score course that involved some 62 scattered, unmanned locations. He showed us the "flight plans" filed by all the teams. These were black-and-white reduced size maps of the venue, with the teams' intended routes and loops marked. He explained that these could assist in speeding a search if a team didn't get back on time. He also used them on a display string at the end of the event so that all teams could compare routes taken. I made a copy of Team 12's (the suspect's) route plan onto a big map. Looking at team 13's plan, Michael Aylott and Ben Baldwin's, I saw there was little correspondence. Team 12's loop one was first southeast, followed by loop two north, and then east, while Team 13 did about the opposite. Something made me copy Team 13's route, too.

Geoff said the terrain was mostly what we'd seen driving in – open forest, rolling hills, many small streams, with lots of old gold mines with unblocked entrances and dangerous holes around. He told us about something unusual on the eastern part of the map, from near here over to control 102. The vetters had to replace two controls, which they'd found yesterday torn down and balled up, plus three of the event directional signs, which had been tossed into the bush. He suspected there must be just some kids around vandalizing, although there was no sign of them.

Gordy said with a grin, "Wrong, mate, it's just the yowie having fun! Or, perhaps not liking humans hanging stuff in his living room. Then again, there's that old sherpa saying from Tibet: 'There is a Yeti in the back of everyone's mind; only the blessed are not haunted by it.'"

I asked what a vetter was. Geoff explained in detail about Setters and Vetters. He said it took weeks to insure that all the 60-some controls were properly set per the issued map. The Vetters inspected the control bags already in place using just the final map and description sheet, and made sure everything was right just before the event started. Rogainers expected good courses, and appreciated hard-to-achieve perfection. He said in ten years of running rogaines, he'd personally set only one control wrong out of over 1000, and had never heard the end of it from his friends! Seems it was a water control at a mapped road junction.

While we waited for the first teams to loop back in for dinner, we had coffee and checked with the catering crew on the food service. They were preparing large pots of stew, vegetarian soup, and a potent chili, and had lots of vegetables, fruit, bread, peanut butter, cookies, and cold drinks set up. Kangaroo tail soup was on the menu. Reminded myself to ask and to avoid it. Several big tanks of water with spigots were set up so teams could refill their bottles or Camelbak bladders. Each rogainer carried 64 to 100 ounces (about 2 to 3 liters), enough to last between water control refills.

The head chef Heather Davies said that, in her experience, rogainers consume more than twice what most outdoor sports people eat. Since teams drift back to the Hash House at odd hours from about 5 PM to after midnight, it was a challenge to keep hot food always ready. Many teams ate, then slept or rested Saturday evening; some ate breakfast, went back on the course again, and then ate another big meal after the finish on Sunday noon. A few teams stayed out all night, ate trail mix, energy bars, or whatever they had, and were gluttonous when they finished the 24 hours.

Heather yabbered on that flawless foodservice was an expected part of a good rogaine, second only to accurate placement of all controls. Socializing around the campfire at night and after the rogaine on Sunday were also experiences people treasured. She started to go on about her eating pleasures, and uses of native bush tucker like midyim berries, but I stopped her with, "Just the facts, Ma'am."

Heather offered us some soup just prepared. It was strong, but tasty. I had to ask—it was kangaroo-tail! She said she'd find me the recipe. We paid for our evening meal (they offered it gratis, but we insisted), and said that we might be around tomorrow, too. We set up our tent for the night, and then hung around to try to see the suspects when they came in to eat. We puzzled over when or if to make the arrest.

Gordy went to the truck and brought back something. He said, "Here's a little prezzie—a weapon you might need if we see a yowie." It was a good-sized, Aborigine-made, boomerang. Didn't look very lethal. Gordy was reluctant to demonstrate a throw, but eventually cocked his arm, boomerang almost vertical, end forward, curved side toward his head, and threw it toward the treetops with a strong wrist flip. It sailed in a beautiful half-circle before it crashed into a bush. I told Gordy I might have trouble getting this fearsome weapon home. A neighbor had her carry-on portfolio full of delicate competition boomerangs confiscated by an airline in Boston recently. I said we'd better stick to chess while waiting. He crushed me in 18 moves.

Saturday, 6:30 PM: Team 12 (Taylor and Smith) checked in, and Team 13 (Aylott and Baldwin) shortly thereafter. Kath Smith (my suspect Kim?) grabbed some food, went immediately to their tent, and stayed there. She didn't look familiar. Kurt Taylor (suspect Knut?) sat down to eat near the campfire, and I joined him. I mentioned my visit to his office on Thursday, our interest in investing in the dredging venture, and

Team XV12, Kurt Taylor & Kath Smith (suspects)						solid route on map	Team MV13, Michael Aylott (dead) & Ben Baldwin						dashed route on map
Time	Control	km	rate kph	Tvl. min.	Sign-in time	Actual Sign-in	Time	Control	km	rate kph	Tvl. min.	Sign-in time	Actual Sign-in
18:30	HH	1.2	4	19	18:30	chk'd in 6:30	18:30	HH	2.5	4.1	38	18:35	chk'd in 6:35
19:00	dinner						19:00	dinner					
19:30	lv HH				19:30	saw 7:30 pm	19:30	lv HH				19:30	saw 7:30 pm
20:00	52	1.4	3	29	19:59		20:00	42	1.4	2.2	39	20:09	
20:30	62	2.2	3	45	20:44		20:30	57	1.5	2.2	42	20:51	
21:00							21:00	76	1.2	2.2	34	21:25	
21:30	72	1.8	3	37	21:44		21:30						
22:00							22:00	93	2.2	2.2	61	22:26	
22:30	90	2.3	3	47	22:31		22:30						
23:00	30	1.3	2	40	23:11	11:11	23:00	66	1.2	2.2	34	23:00	
23:30	20	1.4	2.5	35	23:46	11:45	23:30	103	1	2.2	43	23:43	
0:00							0:00	56	1.3	2.2	36	12:12 AM	
0:30	60	1.8	2.5	44	0:30	12:29	0:30						time of death+/-
1:00	100	1	2	31	1:00	1:05 *time of deati	1:00	92	1.4	2.2	39	1:03 actual	1:05-1:15
1:30	50	1	2	31	1:32	1:33	1:30						
2:00	80	1.8	2	55	2:27		2:00				Baldwin picked up on road		
2:30							2:30	to road	2.5	3.0	51	2:00	arr. @ HH
3:00	51	1.3	2	40	3:07	3:10	3:00	HH	6.5	car 30 kph	14	2:15	
3:30							3:30						
4:00	70	1.8	2	55	4:02		4:00						
5:00	61	1.7	2.2	47	5:19	5:20	5:00						
Time	Control	km	rate kph	Tvl. min.	Sign-in time	Actual Sign-in	Time	Control	km	rate kph	Tvl. min.	Sign-in time	Actual Sign-in

tried to draw him out. His voice did not sound familiar, and nothing about his appearance reminded me of the man I'd met back in 1994. Maybe it was the heavy beard. But he did have a big new-looking Rolex on his left wrist.

Gordy came over, introduced himself, and asked a question or two while eating from a plate piled high with food. I walked over to our truck to grab a coat, as it was getting cold. Kurt moved off and sat with Michael Aylott, and it looked like they were comparing routes on their maps. I wondered if rogaining rules allowed this, since they were on different teams, and the event was still in progress. An unknown woman in dark clothing joined them for a moment, handed each a small bag, and then left carrying a map. A minute or two later they broke up.

Kath Smith, now wearing a shiny white coat, came out of their tent to joint Kurt. Shortly there-after they, and Aylott and his partner Baldwin, picked up their control cards. All then disappeared, going different directions into the bush. I didn't get to hear Kath speak, but her looks had changed a lot if she was the same person I was after. Platinum blonde, shiny white running suit well filled out, and keeping up with Kurt's long-legged strides as they left. She looked the right height compared to Kurt as they disappeared into the dark.

I noted the time: 7:30 PM, was just a few minutes after Ending Evening Nautical Twilight at 7:13 PM, which I knew was when rogainers first needed a light to navigate. Tomorrow's Beginning Morning Nautical Twilight at 5:14 AM usually meant lights could be put away. I remembered my past night outings required both a headlamp and a flashlight to follow trails and avoid stumbling. Also, I noted that most of these Aussie rogainers were going out with small, AA-cell hand lights, and some new LED headlamps. A few teams carried big, 5-D-cell "torches," good for beating off monsters and spotting control markers half a kilometer away.

Gordy and I sat and ate some more, and talked about whether we had enough information to nail the two suspects for extradition. It seemed to Gordy that a good 'solicitor' could kill such an action by arguing for mistaken identity and that everything was a coincidence. And even worse, the restricting fact that theirs was a capital crime (with special circumstances), punishable by death in the USA. He told me the last hanging in this country was in 1967, and he doubted I could even take Osama bin Laden back with me if I found him here. In fact, Queensland was the first state to abolish the death penalty back in the 1920s, so maybe that's why Knut and Kim decided to run there. I thanked him for spoiling my whole day, if not the entire trip!

Saturday, 8:10 PM: About then Gordy also started shivering, and went to the truck to get a coat. I walked down to the portable "dunny" for a break. The organizers had thoughtfully provided some liquid hand cleanser at the outhouse, with no running water around. And a scented candle in a holder on the dunny floor. Returning in the moonless, overcast evening, I thought I heard something behind me—just as a dark car came out of nowhere and just missed me. I stumbled and fell off the road. The car looked familiar. Couldn't get a license number—plate unlighted.

Somewhat shaken, I walked back to inform Gordy. He wasn't at the campfire, but soon returned with a grimace on his face. I told him about the car. He didn't say anything, but told me to come back to the truck with him. He had something in an evidence bag in the back. He told me he had luckily seen some mashed-down grass on the side of our vehicle, and checked underneath. He showed me what he'd found wired to our muffler—a M67 hand grenade, with pin removed and string wound loosely around the safety lever, taped to a bottle of gasoline.

He'd disassembled the grenade. Gordy told me that he'd learned to make similar devices himself in Vietnam during the war, copying the VC. He'd already dusted for fingerprints, but found none. Needless to say, our alertness level or "pucker-factor" went way up! Anyone could have planted the bomb after we got here. It probably would have gone off after we'd driven enough distance on these rough roads to loosen the string. I pictured how Gordy's truck and contents would have looked—nothing left of us but the Roo bar! I began wondering if and when Kurt, or Kath, or maybe even Aylott, had planned this. Maybe after they heard that two "investors" had been making inquiries. But if it was one of them, they must have acted tonight between 7:30 and 8:30, after they reentered the rogaine course.

I got the car license number for Taylor's car from the organizer Costigan, and walked around the car park in the dark until I found it. Checking in the windows, I saw the usual gear. Two partly covered cases caught my eye. I could just make out a logo on the top case. It said Lapua, and I figured by the sizes that these were two Lapua tactical rifles, probably .338. Good enough for going after elephants, armored cars, or yowies. I asked Costigan to move two of his staff cars to block in this vehicle, so I could control their exit I felt stymied. We could do nothing more until the suspects finished the rogaine.

Then I remembered their tent. Thought about the legalities of prowling their tent for about 2 seconds, then did so. Found just spare clothing, swimsuits, some supplies for blisters and sunburn, and an electric lamp hung by a string from the top inside. Used my knife to cut off about 2 inches of the string. Might prove useful for a comparison later. Then I returned to the campfire to visit with the staff members. Two blokes were competing with raucous sounds from bagpipes and a didgeridoo.

They sang me a little ditty that ended:

Up jumped the swagman and sprang into that billabong
"You'll never take me alive," said he
And his ghost may be heard as you pas-ass by that billabong
You'll come a-rogaining matilda with me
Waltzing matilda, waltzing matilda. You'll come a-rogaining matilda with me
And his ghost may be heard as you pas-ass by that billabong
You'll come a-rogaining matilda with me

Sunday, 2:20 AM: We were sleeping in our tent when Costigan woke us to report some business. An accident had occurred at an old mine shaft near control number 92, about 7 kilometers east of the Hash House. A rogainer named Ben Baldwin and his partner Michael Aylott briefly separated shortly after leaving the control. Something happened, and Ben had returned here to get help. We found Ben shivering by the campfire, and asked what had happened. He said that Aylott's illegal radio had rung, he'd answered, then told Ben to rest his knee for a few minutes while he went back to check on something he'd seen at the mineshaft near control 92.

About five minutes later, Ben heard a very loud gunshot, which really scared him. He went limping back and found his partner's smoking Smith and Wesson revolver and his still-lit headlamp near the old mineshaft. He "cooeeee'd" (yelled) for him, but got no answer. Then he said he looked down the mineshaft and saw a body partway down, but unreachable. His first thought was that it was a suicide. So he came hurrying back on his bad knee toward the Hash House to get help. Ben found a staff person, James van Netten, driving the safety circuit that connected the five water drops, told him what had happened, and then they drove back to the Hash House.

By the time two officials got to the mineshaft to confirm this report back by radio, it was too late to stop the rogaine, even if that were possible. Some 90 teams were scattered over 150 sq. km of forested, hilly terrain in this remote part of Victoria. Detective Holman and I went to the death scene, along with the first responding ambulance jeep. The Organizer Geoff Costigan rode with Noel Robinson, a St. John first aide volunteer, in his jeep.

We taped off the area with some engineer tape. Recovered a headlamp, backpack, and a Smith & Wesson Model 629 .44 magnum revolver, 8 3/8 inch barrel. Gordy examined the weapon and remarked, "Now that's a 'fair dinkum' piece, but a lot to carry." I said half-jokingly to Gordy, "It's the newer version of the 'make my day' shootin' iron from an old Clint Eastwood movie. One round fired."

We found Aylott's gear near the mineshaft opening, about 20 meters northeast of control 92. It had a Garmin Rino radio clipped to the top of the backpack. The radio was still on. I looked it over; found it was both a GPS and radio, and that it could transmit the user's position automatically. I later asked Ben Baldwin about it. He claimed not to know how to use any GPS, and that anyway radios and GPSs were illegal during rogaines. He told us that he'd only heard Aylott one time earlier on the radio, near Control 103, but didn't get a chance to ask him about the very short call.

Costigan took me over to the control marker and intention sheet hanging from a tree limb. He said they hung them all like this, about head high, with the 3-sided nylon bag, orange and white, marked with small pieces of reflective tape, and a paper punch hanging down. The intention sheet at this Control 92 showed that the deceased's team, number MV13, had signed in at 1:03 AM.

I checked the sheet for other teams. The next previous team was 30 minutes earlier, and two teams had passed by 25 and 35 minutes after the incident, and before we arrived. It seemed unlikely they would have seen the mineshaft, revolver, or backpack in the dark, some 20 meters off their likely routes. I checked for team 12 on the log. Kurt Taylor and Kath Smith had been here at 2:17 PM Saturday afternoon.

The death looked accidental on its face, but we suspected it was very unlikely that the fall could have occurred where it did without some human hand at work. And what was Aylott shooting at in the dark? There was no blood trail visible anywhere.

Several of us helped an SES team to haul Aylott's body up by ropes from the mineshaft. The victim had an ugly head wound—like from falling a long distance – but he'd been caught by metal structure of old mineshaft elevator sticking out, upside down about 30 feet down the 80 foot or so shaft. No sign of anything above him to cause the head injury. No gunshot wound, unless we'd missed something. His head was still there, mostly together. No blood on the ground visible in the dark. Very suspicious. I retrieved a quick mental picture of what the other murder victim's head had looked like back in 1994. That death was supposed to have been caused by a Sasquatch or a fifty-foot fall at Spiral Butte.

I thought for a moment about a weird scene where Aylott shot at Mrs. Yowie, and Mr. Yowie retaliated and dumped him down the mineshaft. Just a fantasy. We finished taping off the area as a crime scene, left a staff person, Rod Morris, there to guard it and check in still-arriving rogaine teams, and brought the body back to the hash house.

A break in the clouds opened up a view of the starry sky, I looked for familiar constellations and found none. The Southern Cross I'd heard of was just visible. I remembered some night navigation I'd done in the past using the North Star. With guiding stars and a full moon, it seemed to me that rogaining at night could not be that hard. But just then the clouds came back and a cold wind came up.

I found Ben Baldwin at the campfire and asked about the gun. He said Michael had shown it to him just two hours before, and told him it was the right size to bring down a yowie if they ever found one. Ben was worried that Michael was carrying it in his pack on the rogaine against the rules, and even more worried when Michael told him he'd only test-fired it a couple of times. He figured it was more dangerous to them than to any yowie happening by.

Sunday 5:30 AM: A heavy rainstorm hit us just as it got light, soaking us and everything around. I worried about the loss of evidence, tracks, etc., in the area. Nothing we could do, except prepare the body for evacuation to the morgue in Ballarat. Another local police officer, Adrian Singleton arrived, and we shared what we knew so far. We awaited the return of the suspect team, agreeing just to keep them under close surveillance, to question them along with other teams, and to prepare to follow their car, if there was nothing to hold them on.

I remembered the headlamp, and went to our evidence bag to examine it. There was blood on its headband. But the headlamp was on the ground near the mineshaft. So, Aylott was hit by someone or something and was likely either unconscious or dead before his fall. I wondered what he shot at. We checked for fingerprints on the revolver, and found some that seemed likely to match the victim. The lab would make detailed comparisons later. I pulled the two inches of string from my pocket and compared it to the string on the grenade. Looked identical to me.

> There is a Yeti in the back of everyone's mind; only the blessed are not haunted by it.

Sunday, 9 AM: The rainstorm thankfully let up, and the sun broke through to start warming us. At my request, Costigan sent some of his staff by cars with radios out to the northern controls where the Taylor-Smith team should have been last night, per their "flight plan." By radio, we received word that Team 12 had logged in at control 30 at 11:11 PM, control 20 at 11:45 PM, control 60 at 12:29 AM, control 100 at 1:05, control 50 at 1:33, and control 51 at 3:10 AM. I checked this route and timing vs. the "flight plan" map I made up yesterday. Having seen Team 12 Saturday evening, and caught their departure time, those intention sheet entries seemed to match their planned route.

I asked Costigan about the entries on the intention sheets. He explained that teams entered their number, time in, and next control on the sheet on the next available line. Teams recorded their times, which then flow chronologically, and it's not likely that anything on the sheet could be faked. Unless, of course, one team was signing in for itself and another—a conspiracy! But control card punches are a double-check on all that. Teams carry only one control card, which they turn in each time they check into the Hash House. When finished, their card shows hash house times and punched holes in boxes for all controls visited. Teams usually calculate their own scores on the cards after finishing.

I borrowed Gordy's laptop and made up a quick spreadsheet, listing the controls and routes of the suspect team XV12 and the victim's team MV13. I filled it in as I got data from various sources, eating bites of my breakfast while I worked. Some rogainer had cleaned out the last of the big tub of oatmeal. They also ran out of decaf coffee. Completely! I had some of the real stuff, which did help keep my eyes open after only 2 hours sleep last night.

The intention sheet login and Baldwin's recollection of the gunshot seemed to nail down the death to about 1:05-1:15 AM. Another team also heard the gunshot while almost a kilometer distant, and both agreed it happened about 1:15 AM.

We questioned Ben at length about his possible connections with the deceased, the gold dredge business, and incidents during this rogaine. He said he'd practiced with but never rogained with Aylott before. He told us he did have a sizeable stake in the dredge boat venture. However, nothing else came out that pointed to a motive for Baldwin to kill Aylott. His body language and voice showed no signs of lying. He reported seeing what looked like a footprint of a big, bare foot near Control 103. The rainstorm last night had probably washed whatever it was away.

Sunday 10 AM: I wondered if the body was really Michael Aylott, or could there be another switch here, like last time. And what was the actual cause of death? And I remembered the big key man insurance policies – again like the Spiral Butte caper. What bothered me even more was this happening just after the car bomb planting, and my near miss hit-and-runs. I speculated on the likelihood that my two suspects knew or guessed who Gordy and I were. Wished I knew more about the psychological makeup of these miscreants.

Still waiting for Team 12 to finish, I got up and went to measure the corpse's boots. A song line kept repeating in my head: "'You'll never take me alive!' said he."

DUM DE DUM DUM, DUM DE DUM DUM, DUMMMM.

PART IV – Beware Trampling the Midyims!

It was Sunday morning. With the finish time approaching for the Enfield-Jubilee Rogaine, my partner Gordy Holman of the Victorian State Police and I were continuing our questioning of rogainers concerning the suspected murder of Michael Aylott, the business partner of the suspect I'd been tracking. I was now working undercover Down Under, sent by the Sheriff's Office of Yakima County, Washington State, the USA. Pursuing two murderers. My name's NotFriday. I carry a badge, number 714. I'm a cop.

DUM DE DUM DUM, DUM DE DUM DUM, DUMMMM. *(The reader is encouraged to hum the Dragnet theme music now and then throughout this story.)*

I looked again at the map and the spreadsheet on the route and times by location of Kurt Taylor (Knut Phillips?) and Kath Smith (Kim Stark?). It seemed my suspects' team had signed in at controls far removed from the death scene around the time it happened. To double-check on that, Geoff got by radio a list of all teams who might have been near or passed Team 12 between midnight and 2 AM. Three of these teams I questioned later when they arrived at the finish. Two teams confirmed they had seen Taylor and Smith together going south near controls 50 and 51 at about 1:30 and 3 AM. Although they didn't talk, they were recognized by their heights and her peroxide blonde hair seen by their headlamps. We questioned several other teams who'd been near Control 92 around 1 AM. All claimed to have stayed together, and their stated movements checked out with intention sheets and their control card punches. No other team was within one kilometer of Control 92 at 1:15AM.

So, facts seemed to point to a (mythical?) Yowie encounter in the dark, with the victim missing his shot and the yowie dumping him into the mineshaft. Or a murder by partner Ben Baldwin. But not an accidental fall. Or so it appeared.

Sunday, 10:12 AM: When the Taylor-Smith team checked in, the finish crew asked them to compare their actual route to their submitted "flight plan." They modified it to show their route, and posted it with the others on a finish string with their time in and total score. When they left there to eat, I checked on that route, copied it to my working map, and checked with the finish crew. The punches and score on the card had already been checked, and all punches were correct, based on the organizers' master card. I looked at the distance on the map between control 100 and control 92, some 10 kilometers, and muttered a few expletives to myself.

Sunday, 12:30 PM: The rogainers were called together, a brief announcement was made about the accident, and the little koala wooden plaque awards were presented. The reported death of a rogainer

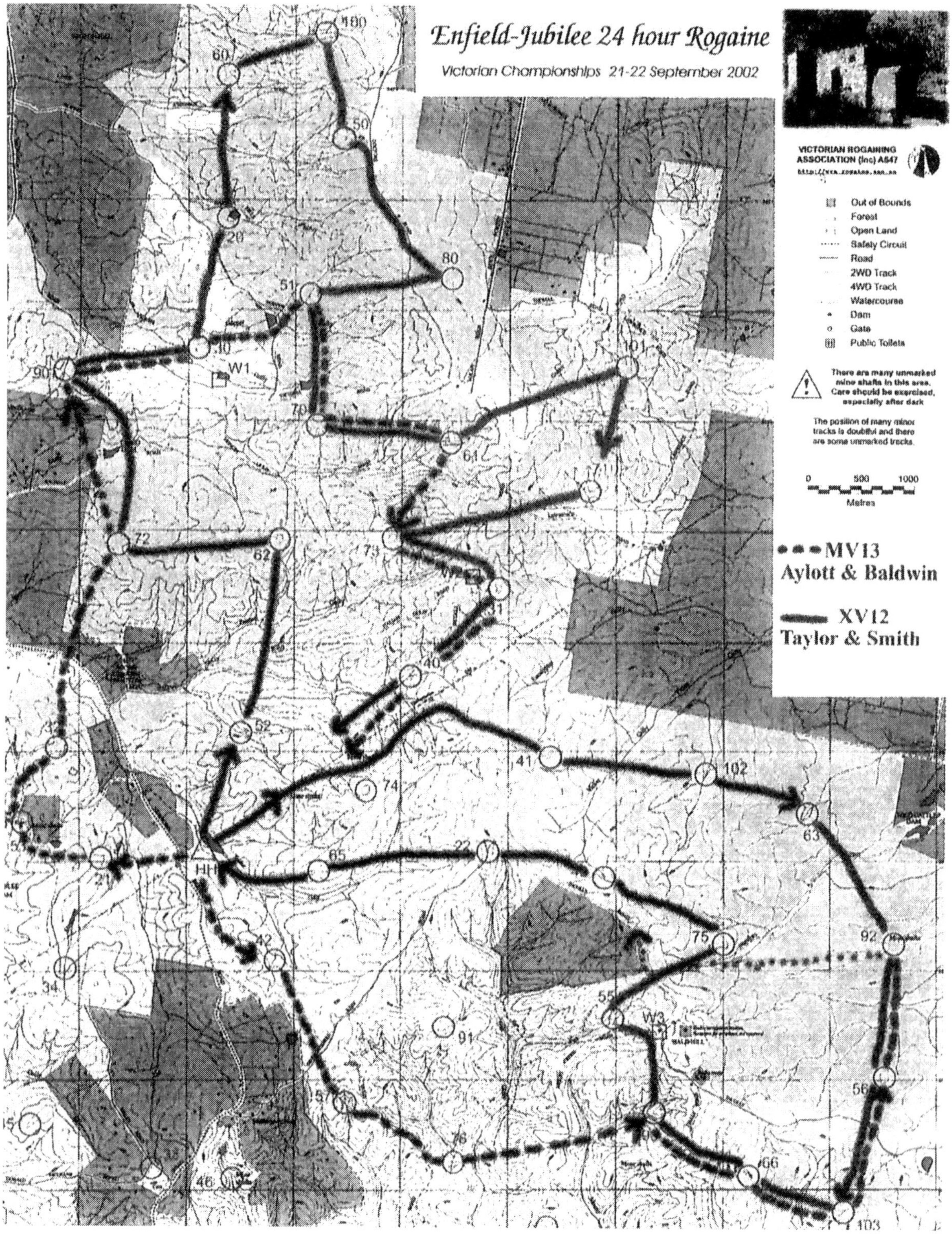
Enfield-Jubilee 24 hour Rogaine
Victorian Championships 21-22 September 2002
VICTORIAN ROGAINING ASSOCIATION (Inc) A547
Out of Bounds
Forest
Open Land
Safety Circuit
Road
2WD Track
4WD Track
Watercourse
Dam
Gate
Public Toilets
There are many unmarked mine shafts in this area. Care should be exercised, especially after dark
The position of many minor tracks is doubtful and there are some unmarked tracks.
0 500 1000
Metres
MV13
Aylott & Baldwin
XV12
Taylor & Smith

was the first ever heard of in Australia, so it put quite a damper on what was normally the highlight of rogaining competitions—the route comparisons and stories of happenings among the teams. Taylor and Smith placed fourth in their Mixed Veteran class, and eighth overall.

We asked several teams to remain for informal inquiries, and released the rest. But not before we checked picture IDs and confirmed addresses, ages, and phone numbers of each participant. Gordy, Geoff, and I questioned Kurt Taylor, Kath Smith, Ben Baldwin, and each of the teams who had seen them between midnight and 2 AM Sunday. We got little more than what we already knew from the intention sheets and our prior meetings.

One team, Mavis Hotchkis and Penny Honeybun, told us that they had been following a team they were sure was Taylor and Smith up north sometime before midnight, between controls 30 and 20, but lost sight of their lights somewhere along there. They remembered recalling then the infamous incident during a rogaine of several years ago. A top team, Nestlecock Arnold and Alasdair Dufty, left the HH after dark, going along a good trail to a control near the edge of the map. They noticed another team's lights following them at their very fast pace in the dark. They decided to ditch that team, if they were actually following illegally. So they deliberately skipped their planned turnoff and went a few hundred meters further, and well off the map then hopped into the bushes with their lights off. Sure enough, the other team passed by, moving fast, and was never seen again until the rogaine was over.

Hotchkis and Honeybun also thought they saw a car moving without lights about then, but figured it was the organizer doing the water drop circuit, and trying not to give away the road location to nearby rogainers.

During the interview with Taylor and Smith, I got a good look at my suspects' feet and shoes. They were still wearing their hiking boots, and their car was still locked. Without a search warrant or any real authority, I was stumped as to how to proceed. I kept hearing that song line in my head, "You'll never take me alive–."

I remembered the beer tent nearby. I invited my two suspects over there to talk some more, and we walked through a patch of muddy ground. I asked Gordy to start the questioning, while I snuck back and quickly measured and photographed the footprints just created. A match! Shoe sizes 16 and 7. Big feet—my big feet! Well, I figured, I don't have any fingerprints or DNA, but I wonder if an Aussie judge will accept the long odds of there being another two people involved in the obscure sport of rogaining, with the right heights, sexes, shoes sizes, a Rolex wearer, about right ages, both from the US or at least not Australian, he right-handed, she very talkative. Or would they argue successfully that they were just two innocent look-alikes? And how about Article 5 of the extradition treaty, where Australia "may" refuse extradition if the US can't guarantee they won't be executed, a penalty not provided for under Australian law?

But what if I can also tie them to the death of Michael Aylott? Both Taylor and Smith insisted they'd been exactly on their planned route, and mentioned seeing other teams up around controls 50 and 51 in the middle of the night. We asked to check out their vehicle. At first they refused, then agreed when we said we'd have to hold them until we could get a search warrant, which could take hours or days.

Our search produced nothing new, except to confirm my guess on the make of the two rifles—.338 Lapuas. No more grenades. No string.

Just then, a crazy laugh echoed across the landscape. I remembered being told about the kookaburra. This crazy bird seemed to be laughing at me.

The suspects behaved normally, eating a big meal after the awards ceremony, and sunning themselves. She wore a tiny bikini—not normal wear for rogainers. Taylor complained about his car being blocked in, and Costigan gave him a line about bad parking by his staff people who were out picking up controls, but he'd try to reach them by radio soon.

I sat down to think and had some more kangaroo-tail soup. Heather told me that kangaroos belong to the Macropodidae family; when translated into English it literally means 'big foot'. We agreed it was a relevant name. I got the recipe.

I left my lunch for a moment and went to our truck—we'd moved it last night to where the finish crew could watch it (avoiding another booby-trap) and got my magnetic chess set, planning to solve a simple little two-move mate problem. My mind must have been on the murder—couldn't solve the puzzle. Walking back, I spotted Kath Smith through the trees, still wearing her bikini, she hesitated just an instant as she passed my unfinished soup bowl. I checked it, and saw what looked like pepper floating on the top. I found an empty can and poured the soup into it to save for testing later. Poisoned bush tucker?

Later that afternoon, after more questioning, the two suspects drank a lot of Foster's, and got quite loud and obnoxious with others. We had a local police officer watch them. Gordy and I reluctantly agreed that we really had nothing solid on our suspects or Ben Baldwin, or anyone else, and would have to release them all. I sat down in defeat, muttering a few more expletives, while Gordy went off to find Costigan to pass the word on release.

Sunday, 4:15 PM: Just then, we got a break, and held everyone in place. We learned that a search and rescue jeep from the State Emergency Services (SES) had just brought Jane Clarke, Taylor and Aylott's secretary, here. Warwick Solnordal, the SES driver, said he understood she had departed the rogaine area last night, got trapped with flash flooding ahead of her on Browns Road, and then when she turned around, she found another flood and washout of the road behind her. She was on high ground between the two spots. Although she saw other cars and waved, no one came to help until late this Sunday afternoon, when a Search and Rescue helicopter flew over, and shortly thereafter, Warwick's SES team arrived in a small powerboat.

While boarding, Jane Clarke asked if someone could bring her bag from the car trunk. Solnordal went to her car, found two bags, and brought both. On the way back to the south side of the flooded area, she told him she had friends at the rogaine, so Warwick brought her to the Hash House. I mentioned to Solnordal that the deceased's backpack had a GPS/Radio locked on, so had been transmitting the deceased's location. He told me he noticed the car had a GPS unit but without a radio in the dash. I asked about her car. He said it was a Toyota Prius, dark blue.

Sunday, 5:05 PM: Gordy and I interviewed Jane Clarke in Costigan's tent, making sure Kurt or Kath didn't see her. Gordy introduced us for the first time as police officers, and explained her rights. We told her we were investigating the death of her boss, Michael Aylott, in a fall last night.

Her shoes were soaked and pant legs wet. Gordy went off and brought back a big towel and some dry socks, and helped her dry off. While very carefully and much too slowly drying her bare feet, he asked her what had happened. She seemed very nervous and upset by her flood ordeal. And still shocked to learn that her other boss, Michael, was killed by a fall into a gold mine shaft. Perhaps too nervous. Gordy nodded at me to draw my attention to a black widow spider tattoo he was rubbing on Jane's ankle. They laughed at some joke he made about the Latrodectus hasselti and one peculiar arachnid eating habit.

Kangaroo Tail Soup

Kangaroo meat has one of the lowest cholesterol levels of all red meat (to serve 100, multiply all ingredients by 50. That's a lot of kangaroos!)

1 kangaroo tail, skinned and cut into joints
olive oil
115g (4 oz) butter
1 large brown onion
1 medium carrot, peeled and chopped
2 stalks celery, chopped
1 large parsnip, chopped
2 bay leaves
pepper, thyme, rosemary
2L (4¼ pints) water
1 teaspoon salt
parsley

Heat the oil in a large saucepan and brown the kangaroo joints, a few at a time. Leave out and drain. Melt the butter and fry the onion. Add carrot, celery, and parsnip and cook for 8 minutes. Place the kangaroo joints into the vegetables; add the bay leaves, pepper, thyme, rosemary, and water. Cover, bring to a boil, then reduce to a simmer, and cook for 3 hours. Season to taste and serve with finely chopped parsley.

Jane relaxed a little. She stated that she brought two small bags here for her bosses last night, ate a "sandy" and then drove back north, the way she had come, back by Browns Road. She told us her destination was a lakeside cabin that Kurt and Kath had about 100 km. north near Kerang. She'd been there once before. It was quite remote, with no phone or neighbors. They were to meet there late tonight, stay for several days hunting the Yowie, and then return to Melbourne.

We asked Jane if it was OK for us to open her bags. She hesitated a few moments, and then agreed. We put a tarp down and spread out the contents of the first bag: two fancy GPS/radio devices, two night infrared lamps, two Russian-made night vision goggles, a big S&W revolver in a holster, a woman's running suit (dull black in color), a black knitted watchcap, and two leather purses, one sealed in plastic. There were some packages of freeze-dried meals, a few utensils, and four six-packs of Foster's beer. Also, some spare ammunition for the revolvers and the rifles. We opened the second bag to find woman's clothing, two books, some shoes, cosmetics, and a platinum blond wig. Jane told us this second bag was hers, and the first one she was just carrying for Kurt and Kath.

I thought for a moment, and then guessed at the events. Bluffing, I said to Jane, "I saw you here last night about 8 PM, driving your car. What was it you gave to Michael and Kurt? She got really scared right then and started trembling, then crying, and started to open up. She said she'd delivered the two S&W revolvers, one to Kurt and one to Michael. She said they'd been purchased for Yowie hunting, and Kurt had called her Saturday morning and told her to bring them here last night. She said she was told that there had been signs of a Yowie around, and in spite of a no-weapons prohibition at the rogaine, they wanted to carry them. She said Kath cautioned her not to be seen by anyone, and to leave quickly. So she'd driven in the last kilometer without lights, and had searched around in the dark until she found them. Then she left quickly to drive north to the cabin.

I asked how she happened to be trapped on Browns Road just 10 kilometers north of the Hash House, at six in the morning, since the flooding reportedly didn't get severe there until sometime after midnight. She should have been half-way to Kerang by then. She said she'd stopped to take a nap shortly after leaving the rogaine.

Her body language told me this wasn't the whole story. I signaled to Gordy, pointing at the wig, and we began a "good cop, bad cop" interrogation routine. We stressed that this wasn't just a rogaine rule violation, but that she was a suspect in a suspicious death, perhaps a murder.

Jane Clarke began trembling again, sat down, wrapped her arms around herself, and started to talk. She told us she drove to a place somewhere near Control 30 last night, met Kurt and Kath there, put on Kath's white parka and a blond wig they gave her. She went on with Kurt to continue the night rogaine, while Kath slept in the car.

"Oh, God! I can't stand this anymore," she exclaimed. "They told me just to keep quiet if anyone asked – that Kath just needed some rest. But they couldn't have done it, could they? Michael being killed in the fall, I mean. I was with them a good part of the night, before I started driving north again." Jane argued that whatever had happened last night, Kurt and Kath were not involved, since she and they were way over in another part of the area. I asked how she knew where the accident had happened. She said the SES driver heard it over his radio as they drove back here from her car. He showed her on the map he had.

We asked many questions, studied the map, and figured time factors. Jane Clarke repeated her story that she had met Kurt and Kath at about 11 PM near Control 30, put on Kath's white coat and a platinum wig, then hiked with Kurt to a bunch of controls to the north in a loop. Kath said she was going to rest, eat, repair her blisters, and take needed medication. Kath told her she'd drive to a rendezvous place near Control 51 to swap again with Clarke, which they did about 3:30 AM (still dark). I checked my spreadsheet again to see that Kurt and his partner (now Jane) had signed in at seven controls between 11 PM and 3 AM—controls 30, 20, 60, 100, 50, 80, 51.

She remembered passing two or three rogaine teams during that time, but didn't talk to them. Kurt had cautioned her not to speak, saying it was against the rules to help another team.

> "Mankind needs it strange animals, its myths and legends and old tales, in order to objectify man's fears outside of himself where he can fight them with man's courage and man's hope. For man is the strangest animal of all."
> — Borden Deal, *The Cattywampus*

"Yes, and you replacing a member of the team is a violation of ARA Rogaining Rules R9, R10, R12, R15, and R22," Gordy said, "calling for DSQ (disqualification) of the team. But we're concerned with much more than that here."

Jane Clark, hanging her head and looking devastated, said she returned with Kurt Taylor to find the car with Kath sleeping in it near Control 51. She said she gave Kath back her coat, stored the blond wig in her bag in the trunk, and started driving north about 4 AM.

I checked the revolver. It had not been fired recently, and was fully loaded. I figured Kurt had put it back in her car last night. I asked Jane if it was OK to open the two leather purses. She agreed. We found in the first one her passport, driver's license, other ID, and round-trip ticket for next week to Whitehorse, YT, Canada. She was shocked, and said her passport was locked in her office desk when she last saw it. She said she knew nothing about a trip to Whitehorse. She also saw that her driver's license showed a picture that was obviously not her likeness. She produced another license from her purse, and we compared them. Identical, except for the photograph. Looked like Kath Smith wearing glasses. The passport had the same picture. I asked Jane if she ever wore glasses. She said only when she drives, but she broke them last month and hadn't fixed them yet. I thought about the two near hit-and-runs by her Toyota. That explained that.

I pointed out to Jane Clarke that the plane tickets, passport, and other ID seemed meant for Kath Smith, posing as her, to be making a trip soon to the Yukon. "My guess is that your employer was about to terminate your services permanently at the cabin. Your trail, if anyone tried to follow it, would vanish in Whitehorse."

She started trembling again. We then opened the plastic bag containing another leather purse. The purse was very heavy, and dirty on the outside. Felt like another revolver. Carefully opening the zipper, I caught the first few of some lead BBs that spilled out. The purse was filled with lead shot! I examine the outside—could be bloodstains in the dirt. The purse had a leather strap about 12 inches long attached. I tried swinging it—looked like a great blackjack. Jane denied it being her purse and repeated that this second large bag was in the car, but was not hers. She stated that Kurt and Kath gave that bag to her to bring from Melbourne to take to the cabin.

She was still trembling and started weeping, so we left her with Alina Danis, a female officer who had just arrived. Warwick Solnordal drove up just then in Jane's Toyota Prius, just retrieved from the flood zone. It looked undamaged. Gordy and I went over it carefully, and found mostly just some additional food supplies. Gordy found an Enfield-Jubilee rogaine map on the floor. It had a pencil line of what looked like the route Kurt and Kath took. I suspected Kath had left it behind last night. The car had a GPS device in the dash. I wondered if it could store the last car drive taken in its memory.

Sunday, 6:05 PM: Gordy and I looked at each other, nodded agreement that we had all we needed on the suspects for the new murder, and went over to the campfire to find them. The officer on duty there had been eating while setting by their backpacks and coats, but now couldn't see them anywhere. I quickly looked and saw their vehicle still blocked in by the rogaine officials' cars. Another rogaine staff man, Bert Keleman, said he'd just seen them, quite drunk and very noisy, walking down the trail to the nearby lake. That haunting song line popped into my head again: "'You'll never take me alive!' said he."

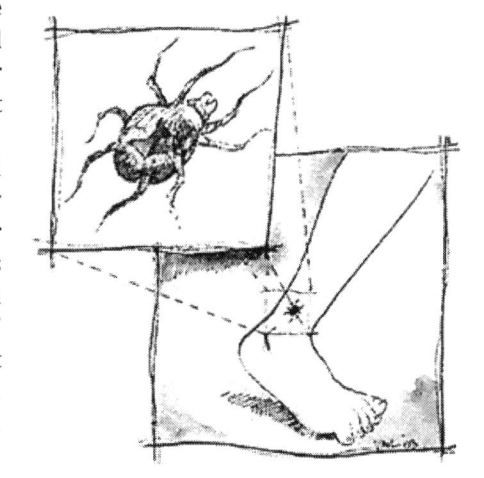

Gordy and I gave chase, and caught a glimpse of them ahead on the forest trail, drinking beer and walking toward a very scenic lake. We were still at some distance, in touch now by radio with the local police officer at the Hash House. They then went out of sight, but we could hear their laughter in the gathering darkness. They vanished among the trees, and when we caught up to where we should see them, they had disappeared. But we had noticed that green shrubbery was disturbed a few meters back near the trail. We backtracked, and spotted a path beaten through the shrubs going into the trees and then into a small meadow full of tasty-looking berries. We continued on the path beaten through the berry bushes.

Gordy said they were midyim, or Austromyrtus dulcis, a bush tucker delicacy. Easily damaged by walking through them, as we were now doing. Searching, but finding nothing in the meadow, or the trees just beyond, we heard loud laughing somewhere ahead of us. We could see glimpses of the beautiful little lake in the dusk through the trees just then.

And then we heard screams—first, a horrible, powerful, unearthly yowl like a baby crying. Then a woman's scream, a man's yell—then, nothing. Nothing but silence! A deadly silence.

Gordy drew his automatic and we started running. I reached for my piece and realized I wasn't carrying. I wished I'd brought the "Dirty Harry" .44 instead of locking it up in Gordy's truck. Or gotten Gordy's hidden spare Glock. Or even the boomerang.

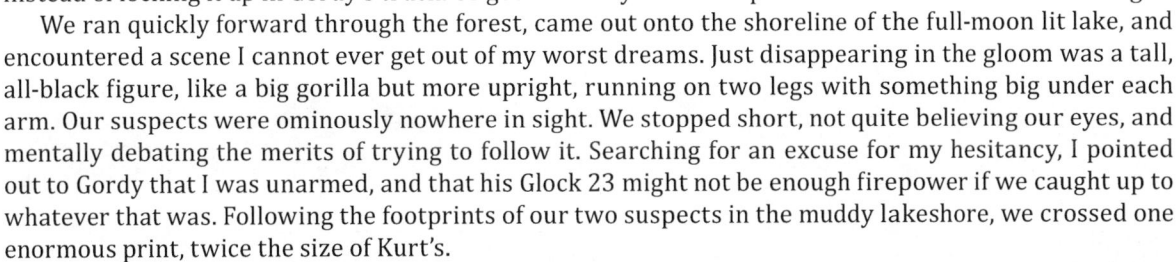

We ran quickly forward through the forest, came out onto the shoreline of the full-moon lit lake, and encountered a scene I cannot ever get out of my worst dreams. Just disappearing in the gloom was a tall, all-black figure, like a big gorilla but more upright, running on two legs with something big under each arm. Our suspects were ominously nowhere in sight. We stopped short, not quite believing our eyes, and mentally debating the merits of trying to follow it. Searching for an excuse for my hesitancy, I pointed out to Gordy that I was unarmed, and that his Glock 23 might not be enough firepower if we caught up to whatever that was. Following the footprints of our two suspects in the muddy lakeshore, we crossed one enormous print, twice the size of Kurt's.

Then Gordy swore loudly, and ran a few steps ahead. He holstered his pistol and peered into the water.

"Mate, looks like your case is done and closed—you've caught your two bigfeet. Whatever that was, it didn't like the midyim being trampled!"

I walked up to peer over his shoulder at a gory sight—a jumble of things cast aside in the water. They consisted mostly of four boots with REI labels, looking about right for the tracks we'd just been following. Crushed midyim berries in the treads. But the boots, size markings 16 and 7, were not empty. Projecting horribly from each was a stump of bloody flesh and leg bones. The bones were shattered as if they'd been twisted off. A trail of blood and a few enormous bare footprints led away.

I told Gordy he was right. "I'm done, case closed!"

DUM DE DUM DUM, DUM DE DUM DUM, DUMMMM.

PART V – The Final Chapter: Big Red Ends It

It was Sunday evening. The Enfield-Jubilee Rogaine in Australia was over, and three deaths had occurred. Gordy Holman of the Victorian State Police and Joe were heading home, having seen the suspects (and the likely killers of Michael Aylott), Kurt Taylor and Kath Smith, dismembered by a Yowie. That's Sgt. Joe NotFriday. He carries a badge, number 714. He's a cop.

DUM DE DUM DUM, DUM DE DUM DUM, DUMMMM. *(The reader is encouraged to hum the Dragnet theme music now and then throughout this story.)*

Sunday, 9 PM: Gordon Holman and Joe NotFriday were heading back to Melbourne, speeding as usual, having left the local police to tidy up the scene at the rogaine. Three deaths, one a murder and two by a Yowie attack. Kurt Taylor (Knut Phillips) and Kath Smith (Kim Stark), previously implicated in at least three murders back in the U.S., were no longer a menace to society. No lengthy extradition to undergo.

Joe's mind was already on his return trip home. He remembered he'd left Seattle on a Thursday and arrived in Melbourne on a Saturday—not Friday. He'd been amused about the coincidence of that and his own name. Now he'd gain the day back, and have time to write up his report on this fantastic Australian pursuit, an unbelievable rogaining misadventure.

Gordy remarked that this drive home was the most dangerous part of any rogaine, with drivers having been up all night, just finishing a tough 24-hour event, and then eating a heavy meal. Joe handed him his cup of strong coffee for another sip. Gordy observed that while the murder case in Washington State may be resolved, courtesy of the Yowie, he still had work to do on the missing bodies and the Aylott murder.

Joe asked, "What specifically?"

Gordy replied, "Well, mate, the SES is gearing up right now to start the search for the two bodies and the Yowie, or whatever it was we saw. A creature that can run off carrying about 160 kilograms, or 350 pounds, of dead weight under its arms is not something I particularly want to catch. The Victorian SES team is getting big elephant guns, a few expert trackers and hunters, and night vision equipment together right now. And I'm ordering tomorrow a couple of test versions of the new .500 S&W Magnum revolver. Dirty Harry would be envious — it has three times the power of his old "make my day" peashooter.

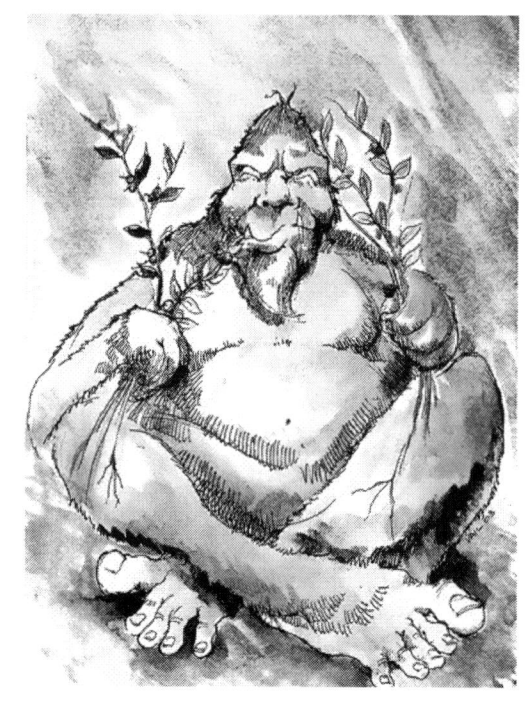

"But no worries, mate. After over 100 years of reported sightings and even older aboriginal oral histories of the same creature, I don't expect we'll find any sign of either the Yowie or the remains of Taylor and Smith,"

Gordy went on to say he'd have to trace the forged passport and the other faked ID, try to find where the grenade came from, and who bought the many other items now in evidence.

Joe snickered and replied, "Yeah, mate, looks like lots of good reasons for you to hang around that black widow tattoo for quite a while."

Gordy suddenly straightened up and said, "Speaking of whom – looks like Jane Clarke's car up ahead. I've just remembered something." He smiled broadly, turned on his flashers, and sped up even faster.

Jane Clarke was driving back home to Melbourne. She was happily singing the new words to "Waltzing Matilda" she'd just learned:

Waltzing matilda, waltzing matilda
You 'll come rogaining matilda with me
And his ghost may be heard
as you pass by that billabong
You'll come rogaining matilda with me

> "Give exceeding thanks for the mystery which remains a mystery still–the veil that hides you from the infinite, which it possible for you to believe in what you cannot see."
> — Robert Nathan

She wondered if those two detectives were now ghosts or might have survived the bomb she'd planted in their vehicle. Jane also pondered what they would do if they lived and found out that she was on that ten million dollar insurance policy as a contingent beneficiary. She thought her plan couldn't have worked better. Kurt and Kath had been implicated in Michael Aylott's death, and her own alibi had held up. Her practicing driving with just the night goggles and no lights had paid off. The radios with GPS transmissions had helped her meet Aylott at the mineshaft, clobber him, and dump him in. Firing the revolver at a bogus Yowie established the time of death.

Jane thanked the Yowie for saving her the trouble of staging Kurt and Kath's self-defense shooting deaths that she'd planned up at the cabin. She smiled about the thought that both of those bozos had separately propositioned her to go off with them to Whitehorse after killing the other, ditching their girlfriends, and getting the insurance. Neither Kurt nor Michael had bothered to ask her if she might like it there.

She mused to herself, "But maybe I will make that trip to Whitehorse for several months until everyone forgets it all, and the insurance pays off. Hummm – ten, maybe even 20 million if they agreed to double indemnity. I could pay a sharp solicitor a huge fee to get that! Then back to Sydney and Bondi Beach for a permanent tan!"

Jane snapped back to reality when she glanced at her rear view mirror and saw the flashing lights of a police car. Looked like the Toyota truck of Gordy and that Yank cop NotFriday. She panicked and stomped on the gas, passing a big three-trailer road-train. She was cursing her luck that the grenade hadn't finished them when, suddenly, a Big Red boomer was right in front of her. Her little car's windshield was insufficient protection from the bounding 200-pound kangaroo.

Gordon Holman and Joe NotFriday were there in an instant. There was nothing for them to do but call the coroner. Gordy was heartbroken and devastated. He'd just wanted to catch up to her and remind her of their date for a Foster's at the pub in Melbourne.

DUM DE DUM DUM, DUM DE DUM DUM, DUMMMM.

The story you've just read is not true. The names have been changed and scrambled to protect the innocent, who sometimes rogaine. Any resemblance to real persons or creatures living, mythical, or dead, is purely coincidental. Some of the contributors were Mac MacDonald, Carl Moore, Donna Fluegel, Neil Phillips, Rod Phillips, Ken Lew, Don Atkinson, and Chris Solnordal. A Rogaining Excuse T-shirt was sent to Sue Clarke, the best interactive contributor. And, many thanks to Rich Vail for his amazing artwork.

ORIENTEERING CONTROL SIGNAGE

> # WARNING! ELECTROMAGNETIC RADIATION
>
> Do not touch or disturb. 50% of this fixture consists of material which exhibits electromagnetic radiation in the wavelengths 5800-6200 angstroms.
>
> Event now in progress—do not remove or disturb.
> If found on ground or removed from park, notify:
> Sammamish Orienteering Club   Call (206) 555-0154

These tags were added to the Sammamish Orienteering Club controls with the hope that it kept random people from messing with them. Visible light ranges from about 4,000 angstroms to 7,000 angstroms. Anything orange, like the bottom right triangle on an orienteering control, exhibits electromagnetic radiation in the wavelengths 5800-6200 angstroms. Any guesses what the other 50% of the fixture consisted of?

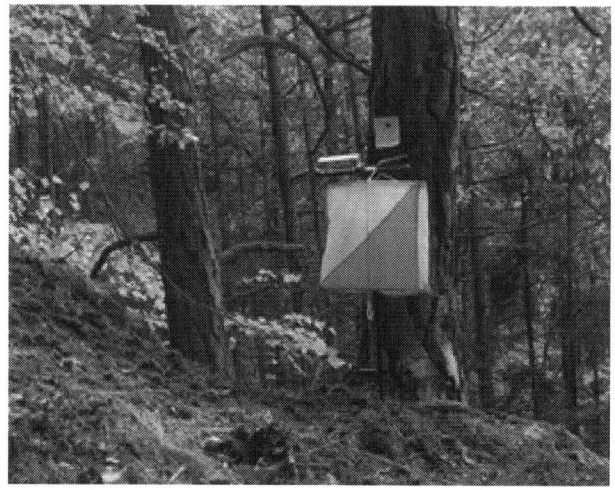

These tags were first used around 1993.

OLYMPIC SIMULTANEOUS

While visiting the Chess Olympics in Nice, France, in 1974, my two sons (ages 11 and 8) and I played in a simultaneous against Antonio Rocha, FIDE rating 2315, the manager of the Brazilian chess team. Even with 27 fellow players, it was a fun game for a Class C player, what with the excitement of the Olympic surroundings and my sons enthusiastic play. Several Frenchmen, anxious to participate in the simultaneous, kept checking the boys' entry tickets, not believing they were bona fide participants. The Ruy Lopez, which Rocha used on most boards, went quickly to the point where I accepted the offered e pawn.

RUY LOPEZ

Antonio Rocha   Bob Reddick

1.e4 e5 2.Nf3 Nc6 3.Bb5 a6 4.Ba4 b5 5.Bb3 Nf6 6.0-0 Nxe4?

The reasons for not accepting this pawn were unclear to me.

7.d4 Bd6? 8.dxe5 Nxe5 9.Nxe5 Bxe5 10.Qd5

His move should have been obvious, but I had not foreseen that I would suddenly be threatened with mate and have three pieces en prise. Some desperate expedient had to be found soon, as Rocha was moving around rapidly, with minimum time at each board.

10...Bxh2+ 11.Kxh2 Qh4+ 12.Kg1 0-0

This prevented the mate, leaving the Knight protected and the Queen developed, although the Rook is lost.

13.Qxa8 c6

My opponent looked me in the eye, smiled, but hesitated with the Queen hovering over b8 before moving. He feared a trap I did not have!

14.Qa7 d5

14...c5 would have delayed the White Queen's return to the scene of action, but I feared for the Knight's safety.

15.Qe3 Re8

Another masked (but empty) threat to the Queen.

16.Qf4

Threatening a Queen exchange; but now I had hope, for his Queen's activity had been at the expense of development. My next move had a synergistic feature–it permitted a fork that was a trap for my busy, traveling opponent. Would he fall into it? My sons were losing, too, but were not so far behind as I was at this point.

16...Bg4 17.f3

The trap was sprung! I looked with disbelief at the square he had left unguarded.

17...Ng3?

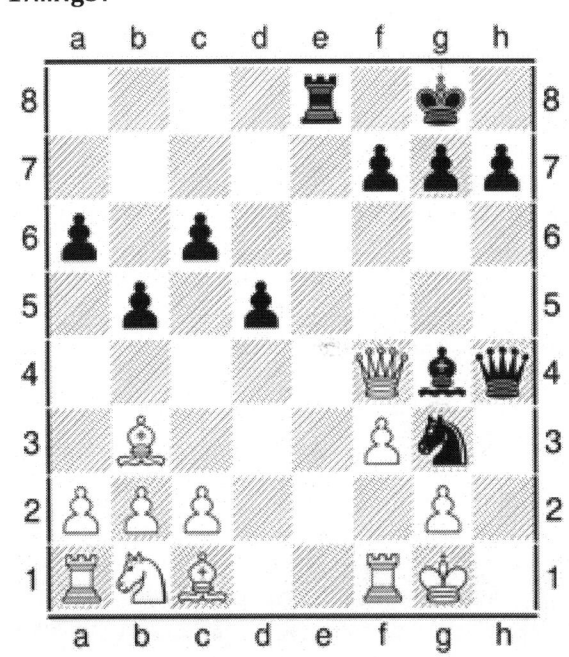

18.fxg4

Two spectators and a fellow player almost broke my arm trying to get me to play 18...Qh1+ instead of...

18...Ne2#

(18...Qh1+, however, also leads to mate: 19.Kf2 Re2+ 20.Kxg3 Rxg2+ 21.Kf3 Qh3+ 22.Qg3 Qxg3#.)

Mr. Rocha, a fine gentleman and a good sport, autographed my score of his only loss of the day.

[My son, 46 years after the fact, notes that 18.Nc3 saves the day for Mr. Rocha!]

Published in *Chess Life & Review* July 1976 in the Reader's Showcase.

NETTLES IN THE KNEES I

Thoughts, recollections, and lessons learned by a novice orienteer during his fifth event, third month:

It's a partly cloudy April morning with almost dry ground and no rain, temperature in the mid-fifties on Mercer Island [WA]. The Sammamish OC event is going well, and I've just escorted my wife and mother through the first half of the novice course. Now to try to really run a course well: all my previous efforts have been walking-learning ones. I decide to run course #3 because Knut Olson says he's going to do it as soon as he finishes his official starter duties. This course is 3.44 km (as the crow flies). Knut's a senior-aged person like me, but also is a nationally ranked orienteer, a bit hampered by a healing tendon. I see that another entrant, Kurt Blakstad (KB), is already at the master map, starting three minutes ahead of me; so I'll be bracketed by experienced people while on the course.

Going for speed, I mark my map from the master in less than forty seconds (making my first nettlesome mistake of placing control #8's number right over an important terrain feature; more on this later). Launching off, running full tilt from the picnic shelter, I approach the stump (control #1) just as KB is leaving it. A few seconds later I'm charging toward rootstock #2, while KB is still standing in the nearby clearing, checking his map. My route is via the easiest dirt trail to a paved street which leads from this park section to the next one south (Pioneer Park). (Second mistake here: my pace was too fast and I had to slow to a walk to catch my breath.) (Third mistake: my shoelace untied and it took 15 seconds to retie it.) I've got a 300-meter lead on KB now, but it'll be hard to hold if I don't keep up a fast pace. I run to the woods and down a trail to my selected-in-advance attack point to get to #2. I carefully pace-count and use my thumb compass—which is no better than a regular Silva, except that I can't drop it! I've dropped and/or lost a number of items in the past outings, including my sweat pants). I hit #2 right on! Great feeling!

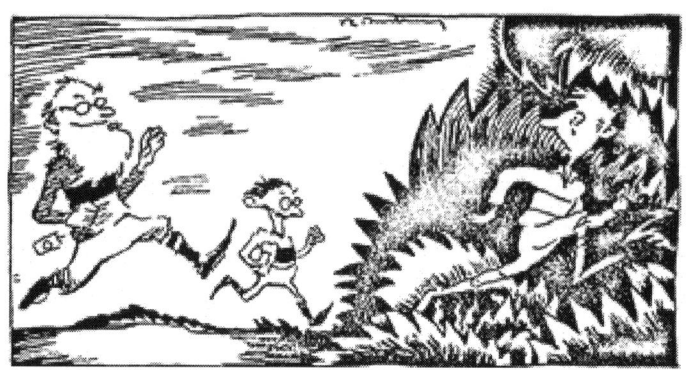

Now to move quickly away, so as not to help anyone see this location. I head for the closest trail going my way to #3. (Poor choice here as a better route would have been directly toward #3, the pit, through semi-open woods with a few nettles, and then using the trail near the end of the route.) (Also, this would have been the time to "aim off".) [Aiming off: purposely aiming to one side of a feature so that despite heading errors, you'll be certain which side of it you'll be on.] Running the trail, I make the next mistake: I fail to visualize the attack point and surroundings to find the pit, and also fail to pace-count and use the compass, resulting in assuming an unmapped "y" in the trail was the trail end, thus losing about 1-1/2 minutes—and a lot of confidence! I recover by identifying two rootstocks, seeing that #3 was due north of them on the map, and walking the compass heading from them to the pit.

Again, I fail to plan my next route carefully, but hastily just return to the easy trail to circle out of this park section to cross the road to the next one. It was a circle that added 175 meters and a minute to my time. The alternate route was shorter, directly through the open woods to the same trail without circling. I then also overrun the earliest place to cross the road by not observing vegetation along the trail carefully. Fred Veler calls this advance picture of what you'd be seeing as you travel, "projecting". I'm trying to learn to do this.

So far, I find the thinking part of this sport to be the most fun, also the most challenging, particularly

Published in *Bearing 315* in 1988. Republished in *Orienteering North America* January 1988.

when I'm fatigued physically from not being in shape for the pace I'm trying to maintain.

Well, now comes the big mistake. I go into the next park section along a trail, pacing to find a junction and then a vague attack point for the stump. The trail junction comes up too soon by my pace count, hut I take it anyway without rechecking. I go a short distance and see no stump, continue on and see that the trail curves left as per the map, launch off into the woods back toward #4, find nothing, divert right to hit the trail to recover. Then I decide to go east away from the location of the control to find an easy-to-identify trail junction on the left to guide back on. After 150 meters, I see by the map and trail bend (checked by my compass) that I'm way beyond the sought junction. I reverse, running to locate it. Doing so, I pace to find a carefully chosen new attack point and as I get there, KB emerges from the woods. Control #4, a stump, is found at last! (I lost 5-1/2 minutes and traveled 500 meters extra while wandering—not "lost"—we orienteers are never lost–it's just the features and controls that are temporarily misplaced.)

Seeing that KB has gone east, I now go west, having carefully chosen a route which will take me by my #6 attack point, while aiming directly for #5, a small depression near the trail. I realize I've missed it when the terrain slopes off and the trail starts down. Again, I haven't paced well (going too fast!) and had no precise attack point. I return to a clearing offset slightly south from the trail junction, and head east again parallel to the trail through nettles and brush to try for the depression. Carefully pacing, I stop when it doesn't show, turn left toward the trail I'm paralleling, and run right into the depression. The control flag is tied to a branch lying across the depression (more like a pit), but it looks as if the branch may have broken—for now the marker's bottom is on the ground. You couldn't see this control from more than 2 or 3 meters away, which I understand isn't fair play. But the feature is there, and Dave Enger's map is accurate. I punch and go. (Lost 1.2 minutes here.) Heading fast for the clearing #6, I first encounter Knut and his protege coming from #4. I realize he's caught up 6 to 10 minutes on me, but I'm encouraged by not seeing KB again. I zip down to #6 in a flash, using my pre-selected and preview attack point, two stumps. I always check the control number before punching, although I'm not really sure this is necessary. I know that the location, feature, and area are checked as correct, and no other control marker is visible in the area. Control markers are supposed to be 100 meters apart, if on similar features. *[Ed. note: you should always check.]* (Oh, I'm using my thumb compass on a map folded in my left hand, with the compass oriented on the map pointing toward my next objective, and with the control punch card stapled on the back. No baggy [plastic map case], as I find them bothersome unless in heavy rain). Now on to #7. I hear Knut and the boy approach as I'm leaving, so I've the incentive to move fast. The second shoelace untying occurs now. and I can't run well without retying—another 20 seconds lost.

I hit #7 by carefully pace-counting up a trail from a trail junction, then pacing by a compass bearing into the woods to the stump. But here I've failed again to plan ahead for the next approach. I stand there reading my map, and Knut and partner catch up! I apologize for giving the location (but he needs help?) and take off on a hastily planned beeline through heavy woods toward rootstock #8. Trails were possible, but the longer way around. My route choice proved bad, because I couldn't (or didn't) accurately pace-count, and haven't yet learned to gauge distances by eye as Knut has. (He later estimated a 40-meter distance for me that was within two meters.) Also I mistook the first trail I came across as the second one on the map, so I was off by 70 meters in trying to find #8. Not finding it. and seeing Knut stop behind me on the trail to read the map with his partner, I retreated there. He offered the advice that we were at a small clearing shown on the map. (AH HA! My #8 red number was hastily placed directly on top of this now important feature, and I couldn't see it.) So I take off fast on a slightly off-compass heading. Knut found #8 just before me, and we punched together. Their team then discussed returning to the trail just left. This time I take off through the woods to hit a previously used trail in the general direction of #9 and hit it quickly. I run to the stump, which is very easy, with a simple attack point, short pacing, and no compass needed. Then out, running to Island Crest Drive and north toward #10.

Now, I'm really tired and resume walking again. Knut's team passes easily, using his easy jogging gait. I try it and find it easier to do than running, almost as fast, and certainly faster than the run/walk (pant!

pant!) gaits I've been using. I take a small shortcut at the next corner, and pass them again running, but poop out soon as we re-enter the park. Using two trails I lose a few seconds (but get to stomp a large nettle plant). They beat me to #10, and are soon well out in front to #11. My route to #11 and the finish are routine and uneventful except for being tired and disregarding the remaining nettles enroute: I'm really not up to the traditional flying finish. At this event there isn't one, anyway, since finishers climb a steep bank to the restroom building. I finish in second place in 60 minutes 23 seconds—with my third loose shoelace!

Since this meet, I've found it very instructive to go over my mistakes, route selections, attack points, gait and timing, and equipment problems. Supposedly, good athletes in skill sports can do some of their best training in an easy chair (a good place for knees to recover from welts) just planning and visualizing in their minds the correct form, techniques, and strategies to use in their future event. Along with the nettles, the nettlesome problems of optimizing the attack on the course while on the move are the most demanding, and the most fun, in Orienteering. I hope that this novice's musings may help you in your efforts to excel in this challenging sport, or perhaps, just help you get back in time for pizza!

QUIZ ON "NETTLES IN THE KNEES"
Arrange in order of importance the following 14 factors that led to time delays on that course:
( ) EQUIPMENT PROBLEMS
( ) ROUTE PLANNING
( ) ROUTE FINDING
( ) PLANNING ATTACK POINTS
( ) FINDING ATTACK POINTS
( ) TERRAIN APPRECIATION ENROUTE
( ) MENTAL VIEW OF CONTROL AREA IN ADVANCE
( ) COMPASS READING
( ) MAP READING FOR DETAILS
( ) SPEED ON TRAILS
( ) SPEED TO CONTROL FROM ATTACK POINTS
( ) MAP MARKING OF CONTROL NUMBERS
( ) MENTAL DISTRACTIONS
( ) PACE COUNTING AND DISTANCE ESTIMATING

(Cascade OC editor's note: When I first glanced at this "quiz", my reaction was that it was both impossible and pointless. But the more I thought about it, I realized that it does have a function by causing me to think. These are areas that Bob identified as places where time is lost. One way to look at them is to divide them into several groups and evaluate each one and see what effect it has on your time. Some of these like "speed on trail" are a function of physical ability and can not be changed easily; others like untied shoelaces are easily corrected and will knock off a lot of wasted time. Still others are mental errors and can be corrected through training and concentration. Still, keep a perspective on the purpose of your sport. Not everyone is looking to shave off a second here and there. But one thing is common to both the recreationalist and competitor: both want to have an error-free course. Take some time and find out where you make your mistakes and look for ways to make your Orienteering outing more enjoyable.)

NETTLES IN THE KNEES II – Route Selection

Yes, gentle reader, the Novice Orienteer has been at it again, learning the hard way how to navigate fast in the woods—by actually trying it!

This time, it was Trollhaugen near Stampede Pass in the Cascades east of Seattle. This Cascade Orienteering Club event drew a good turnout from several clubs on a hot, dry June day in this not-so-open forest by the Yakima River. I'd walked around Course 1 with my spouse Pat, a non-runner, and developed an appreciation for the highly detailed and excellently drawn map. Also, an appreciation for the hunger of the mosquitoes, which were having a field day on anyone not moving fast! Course 1's control 5 boulder had its control flag hung high on a branch on the far side of a tree, and not visible from the feature: a poor placement for any level course. So, I had some concern for what I might not find on the long course. But it was perfect, and a great challenge in route-selection! I asked Dave Enger to show me his near-optimum route, since he was the fastest on this course. He admitted to lots of prior knowledge, having done the fieldwork on most of the control areas. Dave's comments are included below.

So with Debbie Newell egging me on at the start, I carefully plotted my course from the master map, making sure I put the numbers and lines in correctly, and doing it all fast. Well, then came my first and most embarrassing mistake–a 180-degree error launch! I unthinkingly took off fast straight ahead down a trail which took me back in sight of the registration shelter–a 100-meter error. So, retraversing the famous Schuh Trail, I zipped back on track, now following Debbie. My route was perfect to an attack point off a trail end, and I even caught up with Debbie here. I try to choose routes that are fast, direct, and end at attack points (easily identifiable), that are within 100 meters of the control. It's very important to choose an easy attack point, otherwise it's like looking for another control!

Mentally working backward from the control feature to the possible attack points, to the possible routes from me to there, I try to choose the best one. What's best? This is a personal judgment based on all your experience. Roads and trails are obvious choices and, according to Fred Veler, trails up to 80% longer than the beeline rough routes are faster. I'd heard and been using +50% as the factor, but this event convinced me of the +80% rule. But be alert to the fact that the resident deer and elk around here were not invited to help in the fieldwork, so this map (and many others) doesn't show some very-runnable game trails!

It was about 1100 meters to #2, and with my poor running endurance, I didn't expect to see speedster Debbie again, but I met her just as she left it as I approached from below up a reentrant (yes, one of those valleys that goes up). I could have approached this control from above (that was Dave's route), which is supposed to provide better visibility, but I've found I can see and follow reentrants better from below; besides, the best attack point was closer via this route. I'd planned to work today on talking to myself out loud, to register the next control feature and its number in my mind, plus the attack point and expected surrounding, then the route selected, and my own evaluation of the best pace to maintain. But I forgot and only did this mentally; I had verbalized this sequence with Pat on Course 1 earlier, and it helped insure that I wasn't just blindly moving ahead (like I did at the Start!).

Route selection to #3 was very tough. This course was apparently planned with the full maximum 4% climb for the optimum route, which is punishing on the legs and lungs. Faced with a mandatory 9 contour-line climb (at 5 meters each), on a hot day up a difficult to run (or walk) underbrush-covered hillside, or taking long roundabout trails with the same or longer climbs but easier grades, I chose the direct (slow) route. Dave Enger chose the direct route also; he expected to encounter a log-hopping hill climb but was surprised to find it more open. Starting first downhill, I made the common mistake of "falling downhill" or dropping more than planned–which led to bisecting a "dry-until-you're-halfway-across" marsh instead of skirting it. A fast-running stream in a deep bed was encountered next, so

Published in *Bearing 315* in 1987.

rock-hopping (they were underwater) provided the bridge. At least my feet were cool!

Now came the dreaded 9-contour hill climb. Going up a tough 35 meter hillside, following game trails and random switchbacks to stay on track, I was amazed to see as I reached the top and the edge of a logging road, my foot was falling exactly on top of a fresh footprint going my way! Fantastic odds on this! Approaching #3, I first crossed the middle of another marsh, much wetter, which I'd planned to bypass, then to a hilltop. I had misread the map here, seeing a formline as a depression. It wasn't there, of course, so I reversed around the hilltop to find where I overshot the boulder. Knut Olson and Dave both passed under #3, losing 30 seconds or so here, too.

Pat Albright and I had a nice visit here, while I collapsed and drank about a quart of water. Used part of my 5 minute, 14 second rest to study the next leg–another very tough route choice! The fiendish course-setter had invoked the options of a 1.9 km route to the right around a big marsh and a "fight forest", a 950 meter one leftward with some trails, or straight thru–on down a steep hillside, into a fight area bordering another swift-running stream, past an old railroad bridge cut, which was only about 810 meters. Well, I chose the shortest, toughest, slowest one, (the best way to learn so you'll NEVER forget!) Dave Enger again chose the same route, but avoided about 20 meters of green fight by running in the stream itself (6-12" deep), a wet but clever route! I did this, too, unintentionally, in the smaller stream to the left, since it was the only passable route thru the "fight" brush.

I met Doug Sprugel at #4, and we set off on different tacks to #5. I chose a quick beeline to the closest trail, then followed a power line clear zone up a trail to a great attack point–a boulder at the trail edge. It was only 50 meters thru woods to hit #5 right on–a great feeling. Then selecting an "above" approach route to #6, I had to climb a steep bank to the Stampede Pass road, then starting walking down it–seemingly worn out. But Doug came jogging by, which inspired me to know I'd beaten him to #5, so I tried to keep up for awhile. But thinking about my slower pace caused me to forget my attack point–I've found that I'm often distracted by seeing others on the course–must try to ignore them (except when they've obviously spotted the marker I've just about given up on finding). Dave had lots of company here too, as his carpool members Dave Lilly and Bob Rein converged from different directions on #6 as he approached. Dave took the lower route here, contouring part of the way.

The route choices to #7 were two–left the long way by roads and trails, or right through not-so-open forest to the railroad tracks. Dave took the route to the tracks and followed them looking for a good point to cross an overgrown narrow marsh; he didn't find one, so just plunged thru. With no good attack point, he missed the control; he relocated via the survey marker on the hilltop. After being on the course now nearly two hours, I decided to experiment by detouring on the road route to pre-check a possible approach to #8 while going for #7. Following an overgrown logging road, I found a great route, and marked it with my soggy red O' shirt and white T-shirt, which were now hanging around my neck. I couldn't resist taking a few moments to arrange them to look like a control marker on a stump.

Then off to #7, a 2-minute water stop, and back again, picking up the cached shirts. Another course error made here; in climbing the east side of the hill to reach the cliff-top, I turned to contour around a thicket and "fell downhill" again instead of staying level. This led to a tough steep hill climb to recover, then on to the #8 marker. Without really studying the route, Dave took the north approach, directly up the steepest cliff-part of the hill. His notes said he was thinking "bad thoughts" about his route choice, and the more southerly route might have been better.

The next route to #9 was an EXPLETIVE DELETED!! Go 650 meters left thru heavy woods, 570 meters right down a steep wooded slope to railroad tracks, or 360 meters straight down the "cliff" to fight thru another streambed with fallen trees to reach another marsh. By now, you know my choice, made after starting to go left. It was "EXPLETIVE DELETED", then over the edge and sliding down the cliff, starting a small avalanche with a basketball-sized boulder tumbling down next to me, and using trees to slide into or grab on the way down. The brushy, overgrown stream produced scalp-cuts and even soggier shoes, but this was getting to be fun! The marsh turned out to be disappointingly bone dry but led directly to the control. Dave chose this same route–and made no comment about its difficulty–EXPERIENCE BREEDS CONTEMPT for Mother Nature!!?

The route to #10 was directly over a 5-contour hill following a power line–I missed the better route to the right around this hill (which Dave took). A minor mistake came next, when I confused the descriptions of #10 and 11, got quickly to 10 and found it to be a boulder, not a clearing edge. It sure felt dumb then to check the clue-sheet and found it correct. Could have seen #11 enroute to #10 but forgot to look (Dave did). I'll usually route-choose to anticipate the next leg when I can, particularly on doglegs like this.

Road route to finish (a looooonnng run-in of nearly 600 meters) brought me in with the next-to-slowest time of the day, which didn't look all that bad! The nettle stings, branch cuts, and mosquito bites all healed within a week! Looking back, this was my best O' event for learning route-selection and general fun so far. Hope I see more of Len Englund's tough course-setting!

NETTLES IN THE KNEES III

The Novice Orienteer has been at it again, learning by experience the things not found in any orienteering manuals thus far encountered. This time it was Brandywine Falls Provincial Park in British Columbia–a beautiful forested park in a rocky mountain valley near Whistler, which is the classiest downhill ski resort in the northwest, in the opinion of my son and many downhill enthusiasts. Brandywine has many unusual features–a large number of small marshes and ponds, very rugged hillsides and rocky cliffs, powerline clear zones populated by house-sized boulders, the main railroad line through the western part of B.C., a cross-country ski trail system, and a picturesque waterfall. My wife Pat and I stayed in our camper at the nearby Cal-Chek campground; others camped right at Brandywine Falls Park during the hot, dry June weekend.

We helped set up the children's string course with George Pugh, the meet director. Pat and I were careful to help locate the string course away from a sharp drop-off near the footbridge, and were watching for root tripping hazards, but were amazed to find the course being run up a steep rocky hillside (more like a cliff) to the forest above. After setting this course, we felt that the coming regular courses would be easy in comparison. We were wrong! Previous experiences in B.C. should have prepared us for the toughness of the top-quality Canadian courses.

My first exposure to the electronic starting clock came at the start here. The home-made clock, used at many B.C. events, produces warning beeps and a start signal, as well as keeping the official time. Setting off from here, I chose a trail bend to launch off for Control #1, which I missed to the north by some 150 meters. I learned later that a trail bend is a poor attack point, since the mapper can rarely get shapes represented precisely on a 1:10,000 scale map. Relocating here to find my position took some time–involving finding a close-by marsh and checking its shape against the map's many marshes in the area. Also encountered here was the fact that the powerline clear zone on the map, which looked so runnable and fast, proved to be much slower going than the forest, since it was full of gigantic boulders which had to be scrambled over.

The course was laid out so that trail running was the long way around, but if you looked carefully, the ski trail cleared areas were fairly fast. Lots of tree branches trimmed off for skiing littered these pathways, which were only partly shown on the map as narrow yellow "rides" through the forest. It takes careful map-reading while running on a hot day to detect these important features enroute.

In trying to maneuver through the forest over numerous small hills and sharp drop-offs, and around several ponds, I found that using a thumb compass, I must constantly recheck my direction, or I'll drift off to one side (usually to the right). There is also a tendency to pass obstructions like heavy brush and small marshes on the same side each time, causing this lateral drift (obviously, you should alternate). On legs of 500 to 1500 meters, this leads to errors of over 100 meters, totally out of sight and touch with the marker location, requiring a lengthy relocation. I need to practice breaking long legs into shorter ones, going from findable feature to findable feature enroute–like a series of attack points. Another way is to learn to use handrails that are not the obvious ones–like vegetation boundaries, water features, and contour changes. These are things that an advanced orienteer naturally spots and checks off mentally, but us novices are still just trying to go in generally the right direction without stumbling over the rocks and roots on the way!

This course had no water point (the Canadians must be camels) but I took with me a Thermos of water which proved priceless on this very hot day. I've since bought a bicycle water bottle with Velcro fastener for a belt mount, which I fill with the modified Dr. Haas-Martina Navratilova drink formula of 1/10 orange juice, 9/10 water (keep very cold until on course), and a pinch of potassium salt (and maybe a dash of that nasty, deadly sodium kind!) [YES, this is the secret formula–do not reveal it to anyone!] I've tried straight orange juice and Gatorade, but both proved much too sweet and gave a sticky aftertaste. They're good

Published in *Bearing 315* in 1987.

after the event. Having water along has been helpful in restoring clear thinking and refreshing the body during these 60 to 120 minute courses, when water should be taken (at least by me) every 15 minutes, and the threat of not finding (or finding dry) the water point (if any) is eliminated. Less worry and dehydration mean better concentration on precise orienteering.

I've also experienced the "press ahead regardless" syndrome on several occasions when the right move was to go back to the last place you knew just where you were, and try a different route. At Brandywine I saw a control with someone at it as I fought through the marshy brush at the narrow neck of a pond. Yelling out to him "Throw me the punch!" produced the reply "You look like you can swim!" Not up to wading across 5 meters of unknown-depth water, I reversed for once, and skirted around the pond.

Later discussing possible routes on this map with Ron Pontius, I learned that one option–going down into a valley and following along a boulder-strewn hillside on a long leg–would have proven disastrous had I chosen it–a long boulder scramble that you couldn't fully predict from the map if you'd not seen the area before. I chose the safer, known, but navigationally difficult route up and down forested hillocks. Later I overshot a tiny pond; relocating to the nearby road allowed me to zero in on this tiny feature with a careful compass-bearing walk-in.

Pat heard from another female on her course that it was most efficiently run by just following a major trail, with short right-angle attacks to pick up each marker, then dog-legging back to the trail. Not what the course-setter had in mind, but very effective, and I've seen advanced orienteers use the same technique. We all know that the straight-line or most obvious route is not necessarily the fastest, and often is the most difficult navigationally. I'm very slowly learning to look for better, surer, and hopefully faster routes. In the meantime I'm learning that you must use your eyes a lot to detect on the ground the true nature of the terrain–which the mapmaker often did not or could not fully capture on paper! Marshes can be difficult or easy, unmapped game trails can appear, streams can be hazards or highways, and green "fight" areas can be passed through quickly or can consume much of your energy and enthusiasm in a few yards of desperate struggle.

I learned the next day from Canadian expert Peter Smith (he did the same course in 65:48 vs. my 153:17) a very valuable trick He said that if you suspect that there will be any water hazards on your course–streams, wet gullies, marshes, etc.–go immediately before the start and wade through one!! Once your feet get wet, you'll be mentally prepared for, and not subconsciously deterred by any water challenges in your way. Pat and I also learned here that those cross-ticks on the powerlines on the map are not arbitrarily placed, but show the exact location of the transmission towers or poles, which are highly visible reference points.

Be warned, dear reader, that this Novice Orienteer, now running courses with wet feet, flopping water bottle, and a head full of untried advanced orienteering techniques, may soon move up into the exhilarating world of Intermediate Orienteers, who, I understand, get even more "Nettles in the Knees!"

NETTLES IN THE KNEES IV

First, a confession: This novice in his 9th month of orienteering, and fourth article with this title, just received his first "nettles in the knees" for real at the Lake Tradition meet at Issaquah near Seattle, WA. The title came from my first meet, when the conversation of experienced orienteers included many references to such bodily marks of courage and/or blundering but displayed proudly. Temperature that day was in the low 60's, sunny except in the thick forest, and dead dry.

Second, an apology to two of the three Daves, who patiently waited and worried while I once again experienced the pleasures and pains of this great sport. The third Dave is challenged to run his mapped course (with perfect knowledge) in the recommended 60-80 minutes for an advanced 7.2 KM course. And run it again and again continuously until he makes that time! Hey Dave, I'm at least half-kidding!

Well, here's the blow-by-blow-by-blow of this meet (beginners are cautioned to stop reading here, or proceed at your own risk); hopefully, there are lessons here. Lesson one: when the course planner and the meet director both warn you off the advanced long course, saying it's challenging and difficult, and not vetted, and suggest the shorter one–heed their advice!! I argued with myself for ten minutes while warming up, then another 10 minutes while modeling for photos for a proposed Modern Maturity magazine article. Feeling great after a good run the previous day, I opted for the challenge of the long course, and stapled the long course description sheet on top of the shorter one on my map. Launching off, the first two controls went well, with only minor relocations required. I'm learning to quickly give up on my initial attack when it fails, not wandering around aimlessly looking for the control, but quickly moving out to a known point to attack again, with better compass aiming and pace counting.

The third control was one of those sheer luck ones–330 meters thru woods with no guiding features, then finding the marker before finding the swamp attack point. Quickly going to #4, I came out of the woods onto the edge of a large swampy area, and mistook it as the two connected swamps (now dry) I was looking for. Cutting directly across, I ran into spongy ground, considered going around, saw hikers sitting on a bank at the south end watching me, and decided to plunge ahead so as to not look like a wimp. Blunder of blunders! The ground firmed up nicely, so I sped up–allowing me to plunge up to my crotch in thick, sucking mud. Of course my map, description sheet, punch card and compass were totally soaked in mud.

With difficulty I extracted, circled around the "swamp", found no control, said "Hi!" to the hikers, and asked if they'd seen my plunge. They said yes, but that I had been lucky–a previous orienteer (rumored to be Rick B.), had just been extracted by two others from the same place. They also remarked on my scalp wound, received somewhere back in the woods when a big limb I stepped on had recoiled me up into a low branch. With further search and pacing, it suddenly dawned on me that this "swamp" was actually the much larger lake to the south, which was now bone dry in our 5-month, 50-year record drought. (And this is Seattle??!!) My estimating of size and distance needs lots of work, plus my recall of nature's changes of water features.

Control 5 was perhaps the toughest for a marker in its correct location–I first overshot finding the small trail off the gas pipeline ride; had to pace back from the rocky bluff to the south. Then careful pacing and compass work produced no control! But lots of unmapped debatable dot knolls and lots of vetting tape hanging around. I relocated quickly to the logging road some 200 meters to the south–OK except for the hill climb to it. Then using a sharp bend in the road to set an attack course, paced back again to the same spot from this different angle, but since my pace is much shorter in downhill and log-crossing legs, I added on 20 more paces, and there was the control!! A great feeling of success–I rewarded myself with the last of my water. I noted here that I had been on the course 2 hours and nine minutes, and this was just the half-way point. In my opinion, no course taking more than 45 minutes to walk should be set without at least one water point. This holds for any time of the year, not just hot weather. Most any sports medico will confirm this need.

Published in *Bearing 315* in 1987.

Control 6 was only 200 meters away, but a direct walk there produced only more vetting tape, and lots and lots of unmapped boulders. I decided to relocate to a close by water course, then paced back to find the control between two huge boulders not seen before. Now it was decision time–to go to #7 via trails (estimated at 2200 meters, actually measured at 1900); to go via the direct route through the poorly mapped, slow-run, good visibility forest for 800 meters, or go home to a DNF. I still felt good physically, although out of water–then the final decider came when I heard the crashing of limbs and footsteps–the sounds of another approaching orienteer! Or was it a deer? But I figured what the hell–go for it! I chose the direct route, offset to meet the trail to the east of my control for a good attack point. I had to cross 5 water courses at 50 to 200-meter intervals, so carefully pace-counted, watched contours and compass, and checked off mentally each one. Hit the water course and trail crossing east of #7 right on, another remarkable feat for me, giving a great feeling of successful precision orienteering. Immediately following, of course, came the return to reality as the short attack from the trail bend to the water course and down it produced nothing. Sob! I moved immediately and fast to the major trail, relocated west to the old bus, paced back to check off each side trail to find the trail to the water course, and hit the marker!

Don't ever bet your socks on the detailed accuracy of the map–between Mother Nature, mappers, cartographers, and woodcutters clearing growth, Murphy's Law will prevail on your courses. Unmapped water courses and a map error here had thrown me off. Well, again time to head back, or try one more? My thoughts were all on control-finding now, not what the rest of the world was up to, so I started running again after nearly 100 consecutive minutes of brush-crawling. My route to #8 was by trail to a nearby power-line tower, then thru a narrow green fight area (easy) into a rough open land/slow forest area toward the control (impossible). The control was backed up by a freeway right-of-way fenceline in the green for a backstop, so I figured that if the course-setter could get there, so could I, and not miss it! [Little did I know that he couldn't–and didn't!!] Downed trees and slash in the rough open made it impassable, and I was seized with severe back-of-thigh leg cramps here.

Deciding at last to DNF, I tried to circle around the green to head back. Hit a game trail which took me to a vegetation boundary just 120 meters from #8's supposed location. By then the cramps went away, so of course I couldn't resist going for it! Ran into vines and thorns, and had my glasses flung off into a dense clump of berry vines. This was my first real chance to use the special features of Joseph Huberman's new Treklite O' shirt I was testing out. I used the hand guard and arm patch to sweep through the thorny vines to uncover the glasses–another 5 minutes gone. Lesson here is to tie a fluorescent orange tape to the glasses or keep my soggy headband in place to retain them. I don't like the regular elastic strap around the head, unless I expect to be upside down! Shortly thereafter my empty water bottle got ripped off its Velcro fastener undetected, by a vine, while others were ganging up to carve me up thru my "thorn-proof" pants and gaiters. I even tried dropping down the hillside to work thru the forest, but it was also impossible. Finally, struggled back to the power line ride, ready to give up, and there hung #427 on no feature in the ride! My mud-soaked clue-sheet was somewhat illegible, but it sure looked like #427, not 421 on it. It was 220 meters off the mapped spot.

After many, many bad thoughts passed about the ancestry and worth of the course setters, it occurred to me that the control was here for the same reason I was–there was just no way to get to the mapped place! I then walked a few meters over to look down the steeply forested bank to the freeway, wondering how a bridge could possibly be down there across a creek, mapped as going from noplace to noplace at right angles to the freeway. Curiosity overcame good sense, and still sure that someone was behind me on this course, I plunged downward eight 5-meter contours to find this "bridge". Sure enough, this fascinating old two-lane concrete bridge stood alone, marking the path of the old Snoqualmie Pass highway, probably. Worth the trip down? Certainly, but not worth the 8-contour climb back up thru steep heavy forest and near-cliff banks. Careful map-reading produced a likely route through a gate, if open, up a grassy gas pipeline ride bank some 300 meters west along the freeway. I climbed a fence and hopped the guard-wall to run along the freeway shoulder, probably scaring the passing motorists, and started pace-counting to find the fence.

First obvious sign of mental fatigue came here, (I know, you detected it many controls ago!) when I planned to count 120 paces running for about 240 meters, and switched that to 120 meters instead. Took an extra minute to sort that out when the gate didn't appear, then on to pass through the thankfully open gate to climb the slick, steep, but grassy slope for those 8, no–now 9 contours. Approaching total exhaustion, I saw that my route back logically passed by the remaining four controls, so of course I rationalized that if they're still there I'm going for them. The next two were easy, comparatively, but number 12 didn't show in two tries, but the two pits did, so I figured marker pickup was in process, along with the attempts to locate my body! Number 13 was also missing, which we had used for the earlier photo session.

Again, Dave, Dave, and Dave, I apologize for the 5 hours, 11 minutes for an actual 13.98 km. on the course, and the concern I caused. It was a small satisfaction to learn that everyone else had DNF'd, so I finally got a **FIRST**PLACE**! But never again the Long Advanced! I promise!

NETTLES IN THE KNEES V – Night Orienteering

"It was a dark and stormy night ..." Well, not exactly. Wonderwood Park in Lacey near Olympia, Woodland Park in Seattle, and Tenalquot at Ft. Lewis recently gave this Novice Orienteer his first exposures to night orienteering. It's really different, fun, and worthwhile–to give you confidence in your navigation abilities in tough conditions. The Nisqually Orienteering Club's Jack-O'-Lantern event went pretty well on Hallowe'en, and the courses that Jim Andersen, Don DeWees and I planned worked pretty well. Gary McCausland corrected the placement on one control on the short course–it was behind a stump (headless tree!) and was just too hard to see for beginners. Another control feature was not only difficult to find, it was very difficult to locate to even place the control, requiring pace-counting on azimuths from three directions to locate the mapped stump–which was overgrown with fresh sprouts. All control markers were reflectorized, and a bag of candy hung nearby, plus the short course features had Hallowe'en decorative figures on them–so there were several items for flashlights to pick out (until the Troll bagged your flashlight!).

I used a headlamp there in testing the course–a peculiarity of this REI headlamp was a depth-perception problem first noted in Ape Cave on Mt. St. Helens, when I kept stumbling over small rocky spots in the cave that others passed over without problems. The solution was to tape over the bottom perimeter of the headlamp lens, which kept the scattered light from hitting my glasses–which had destroyed my depth perception in the dark. I used a second small flashlight to help illuminate the trail, the map, and to search for features while navigating. Seems a good idea to have a second light as backup, anyway.

The COC's Woodland Park meet was my first running experience in Night O'. I had run at this park once before and had much trouble in doing the photo memory course. Photos of features with controls were at the start, along with an unmarked map. Participants had to memorize and go with just a description sheet and punch card to try to locate the features. I had to return to the start about 4 times to restudy the photos and the map when memory faded. That experience allowed me to run this short night course in a very good time, hitting most controls with no need for pace counting or a compass. I then rested and watered up and let most of the others finish the long course, while I plotted what to do next.

The long course description sheet looked more challenging–with those shallow reentrants that I'm notoriously bad at. Mike Schuh had taken up my challenge at the aforementioned Jack-O'-Lantern meet to do the Goblin's Delight course–running Course 1 with no flashlight, after having finished Course 2 (3 common controls). He carried that one further and did it from memory with no map and finished in great form! Well, you know what I was thinking: Put headlamp away–put flashlight and map in pocket just in case, and start memorizing the description sheet for Mike's course!

Looking at the overcast sky, I noted that the Seattle lights provided a skyglow enough to distinguish pathways from grass under the trees, except where the fall leaves concealed everything. I had seen that the park perimeter had enough streetlights, tennis court lights, and passing traffic to give some illumination. I also noted that there were no controls common with the short course, and that I had encountered almost no limbs or underbrush unexpectedly (what, no nettles?!) in my previous run. Decision–go for it! (An experience while checking out a String Course location at Tenalquot the following week revealed how easy it is to get off course or turned around in dark woods when you don't use a compass. It's clear that lost people are properly advised to stop and make camp after dark!).

With about a 7 PM start time (very dark!), I spent about 4 minutes studying the master map, trying to not only memorize the controls and my optimum route to them all, but also looking for potential errors as Peter Gagarin advises. I noted that the marsh was in quotes on the description sheet, and that one reentrant branched near the top. It was also nice to see that several controls were on spot features like light poles that would require no prolonged searching.

Published in *Bearing 315* in 1987.

So, I launched off, lightless, mapless, into the park. The first copse of trees feature was found quickly, but a circuit of its north perimeter produced no control. These were small 8 oz. juice cans with reflector tape around them, usually hung on a tree-limb with white string. I started to go to a smaller group of spaced trees to the north, when I saw three flashlights coming from there toward me–other orienteers on the right route? Sure enough, they went to a tree I had just left and lit up the marker hanging high up. Punching in behind them, I noted that the control was almost invisible without a flashlight until you were within about 2 meters–but I also observed that the vertical string showed up more than the can.

The next three controls were easier, although other orienteers helped illuminate the bushes I was searching one-by-one in the saddle. The tough part was trying to find the right place on the control card to make the punch! The "marsh"(?) control was located on a steep hillside, with the only aid to navigation being a nearby road downhill that I bounced off of to locate. A fence corner control, then a hard run brought me to the dreaded reentrant–but now I couldn't remember what the control circle looked like on the map. I swept the reentrant from side to side going up, then took the right fork, and found nothing (but it was very dark). Then I cut across the spur to enter the top of the other fork and found myself right back into the main part again! Very uncertain, I started sweeping up the left fork, finally spotting the white string in a tree. The boulder came next, and the can was seen in silhouette on top of it from a distance, with help from Aurora traffic headlights passing by.

The route to the next tricky reentrant gave a choice of skirting the lighted tennis courts, where I had startled players when I ran wildly by with headlamp blazing on the short course, or over rough open and wooded terrain to beeline to my chosen attack point. I chose the beeline to avoid messing up my night vision with the tennis lights. They still gave enough light that I could make out the rest of my description sheet, which was already nearly forgotten. The reentrant control placement seemed to be much lower down than I remembered from the map, but my sweep-every-bush technique worked, as did my Braille method for finding the card punch position, so I blasted out onto the practice fields to use the fences for handrails to the two power poles.

Reentering the woods in the dark, with no remembered trail to climb up a forested hillside looked forbidding, but a gap showed up when I hit the hillside, and I ran up and right past the dot knoll, the next control. It looked like a bush in the dark, so I searched the larger knoll to the south, finding a marker-like silver Rainier beer can in a tree (empty–too bad!).

Jean Davis caught up with me as I rechecked the bumps to find the dot knoll back the way I came–she had drawn this map back in 1981, and is now back into Orienteering after a long layoff. The last control, a little boulder in the dark, but very near the finish, was almost overran, but the glowing fire at the finish helped me see the can on its top. My now-ritual yelling run-in produced a very good 36:30 time for me, but the best part was finding that map memory is possible and useful, perhaps even for daylight events.

After a great pot-luck get-together at the Millers that night, saying good-bye to Tom Gloor on his return to Switzerland, I drove home listening to Roussel's First Symphony–"Poem of the Forest", almost a theme for Orienteering, which seemed to be a fitting end to a fun evening.

DRAGNET ROGAINE '88

DUM DE DUM DUM.
This is the forest. It was Saturday, May 21. It was hot and sunny in B.C. We were working the day and night watch out of Knutsford Campground near Kamloops. My partner Knut Olson. My name's NotFriday.

A man called—said he'd lost some controls. Seemed somewhat frantic. I asked him where. He said they're somewhere north of here in the woods and rangeland. I asked how many. He said forty, and he was offering a reward for every one found. My partner and I don't work for rewards, I told him, but we'd try to find his controls. We agreed to meet at Lac du Bois out in the forest on Saturday morning to begin the search.

9:00 AM. Knut and I, with Pat Reddick assisting as backup, arrived on the scene early Saturday and cased the area. Looked dry, hot, and forbidding. A lot of others were showing up to assist in the search, too.

10:00 AM. The man, a Mr. Murray Foubister, passed out a few old 1:50,000 government maps to work from, but we all agreed they weren't too reliable. The likely search area covered 125 square kilometers, with lots of ups and downs. About 7600 feet worth of ups, if you happened to choose the optimum route! Most of the others broke down into teams of two, like us, and each team decided to go their own way to try to find the errant controls. At Mr. Foubister's insistence, we all agreed to return with our reports of success or failure not later than noon the next day.

12:00 noon. By noon Saturday everyone was geared up and ready, and we all set out in different directions to begin the quest. Foubister has told us these controls were kind of red and white, and were likely to gravitate to topographical features that were supposedly prominent on the old map. He had set rewards based on how far away, or far up they were from his camp when found. He thought that might motivate some teams to try for the hard ones. He was right.

Well, we found much the same thing that others did—the hard ones were very hard. One control on the SE side of Mt. Wheeler kept itself safe from the prying eyes and the best Orienteering efforts of many experienced team, including the [Scott] Donalds, who spent 4 hours the first day, and again 3 hours on the second to nail it down without success—while novice teams jumped [over] it quickly. Another control's location suckered people off the west edge of the map, where they were lucky to ever return, much less find the right road to the control. Teamwork was very important—Knut and I alternated in route planning and then, while on the move for 22 hours, not-so-silently swearing at the pace and route choices of each other. My partner was also given an impromptu shower when I moved an empty (almost!) water can around as he was refilling our bottles from another can.

10:17 PM. Knut and I tried for one control by sneaking up on it in the dark from one of the four well-stocked water points, some 500 meters up a steep wooded hill. A frog snitch gave away the hidden small pond's location before the quarter moon revealed it, and we nailed the control right on! Returning back down on compass and headlamps, we came back within three meters of our start point!

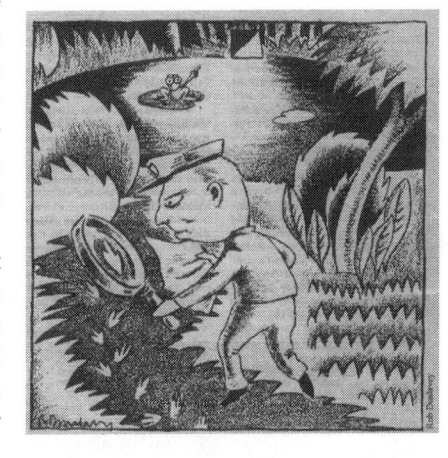

DUM DE DUM DUM.

12:35 AM. Amazed and encouraged with our skill (or was it luck?), we tried to nail #32 from #25 at 1 AM, only one kilometer through the woods and up a steep hill.

1:30 AM. Our headlamps revealed that we were 3/4 way up a rockslide hillside that now became an

Published in *Orienteering North America* July 1988 issue.

unclimbable cliff, and we're too tired to retreat at that point. Our camp consisted of sitting against trees on a steep slope, and wrapping in space blankets for two hours. The clear night gave a beautiful view from our "penthouse" out to the lights of Kamloops some 20 kilometers to the south.

4:00 AM. At first light, starting to shiver in the 5° C (40° F) temperature and light wind, we packed up and made our way down the rocks to re-attack via a road to the east The old logging road shown on the map never appeared, so we circled north to try for #36 at a pond. As the other teams also reported, there were many ponds in that rough neighborhood, and the one we all sought had shrunk up enough to leave a marshy area to its north. The control snuck off from the water to the far end of the marsh and hid in some brush, where only a few could find it after an extensive area search.

7:46 AM. Knut and I had spent the past four hours exploring a good part of Dairy Creek, verifying that old mapped logging roads were no longer despoiling the timbered terrain, and finally returning to the McQueen Lake water point. Reconsidering our find-them-all search pattern, we decided to establish the whereabouts of a gaggle of cheap controls in the hilly rangeland around the base camp. We found the #11 had migrated from the west side to the east top of its knoll, and then moved out of sight of its log-sheet bag. And #6 had moved from the tree on the east side of a hill to a tiny bush hiding next to a big boulder on the top of the hill. In the open terrain these migrations did not help them, as they were still easily captured.

11:17 AM. Approaching the noontime deadline on Sunday, Knut and I wandered back to Foubister's camp—where the other search parties were assembling. No, we didn't bring those controls back with us, but we did give Murray our reports of where they were or weren't, and in return his wife Joan offered up a rustic, plentiful, and delicious meal. We asked her for "just the fact, Ma'am?" She said the earliest teams began dinner about 5 PM, and some returned to eat as late as midnight. Hot porridge was on all night, and first breakfasts were eaten about 4 or 5 and on through about 9 AM. Then returning teams came back for chili and lunch, so we noted that she had been serving searchers almost continuously since Saturday afternoon—a remarkable achievement.

12:10 PM. Interviews with other ROGAlNERs revealed that Amy Loomis and Arnold Kay reluctantly followed a bear cub for a while, keeping a sharp eye out for its mother; an elk and numerous squirrels were spotted by Carl Moore; Shirley Donald found many skeletons of animals; and we all raised many grouse and other birds in our travels. Wildflowers and even orchids were found, and a few geodes, too. Other than minor blisters and a little sun exposure, no one was injured in the line of duty.

1:00 PM. After all reports were in, Foubister gave out his rewards. Top teams won medals from the City of Kamloops, and a few other mementos were collected. The best detective duo were Ross Burnett and Peter Findlay, who found all but one control in about 70 km of searching; Marion McKellar and Amy Shaw, both from Calgary, easily outdid the rest of us for second. Everyone agreed the efforts of the past 24 hours had been a valuable duty and experience, and wished Foubister and his assistants success in future efforts to keep those errant controls in check. Someone asked (a little too late) what ROGAINE stood for, and learned that besides being a commercial hair-restorer, it also means RUGGED OUTDOOR GROUP ACTIVITY INVOLVING NAVIGATION and ENDURANCE, a form of madness originating in Victoria, Australia, back in 1976 or so. A Mr. Andy Newson alerted all of us that he was also having errant control problems in the Ghost River area of Western Alberta, and might need our sleuthing help rogaining in June.

On May 22, in and for the city of Kamloops, Province of British Columbia, Canada, the errant controls were tried and convicted of exacerbation, unauthorized relocation, malingering, and other infamous crimes too ghoulish to relate. The maps were convicted as accessories. They are now serving time in some ROGAINER's closet, probably awaiting the chance to break out for another of these events.

DUM DE DUM DUM, DUMMMM.

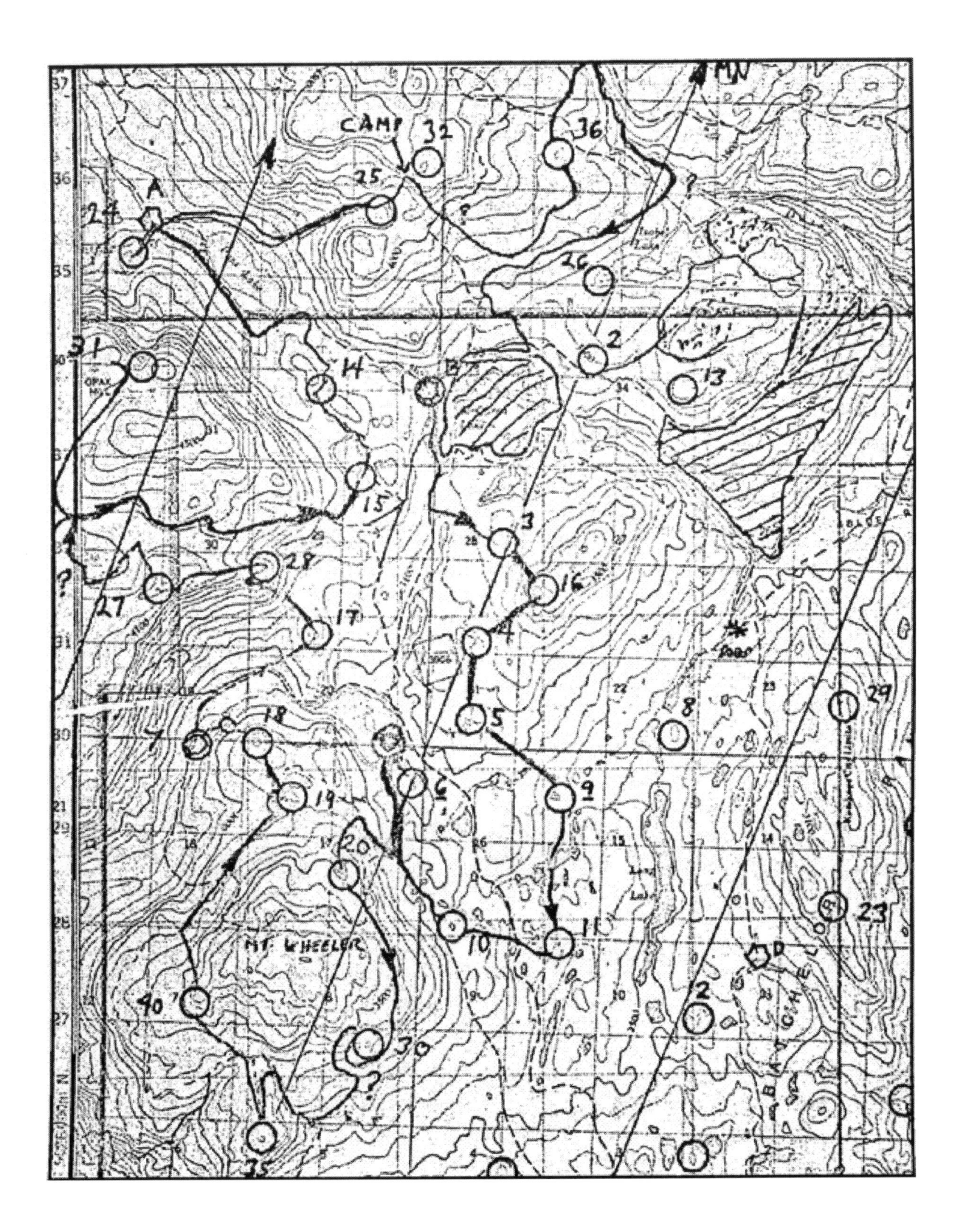

THE (PRE-SWEDISH) HISTORY OF ORIENTEERING

Recent historical research has uncovered some remarkable evidence of the genesis of Orienteering–back before the Swedes "invented" it! Let us return to the [thrilling] days of yesteryear, circa 1904-05 to Washington (no, not the state, the city), where the Secretary of War's Army aide is delivering a message to the White House. He is ushered in to the Oval Office, salutes, and delivers a hand-written note from Mr. Taft.

The President scans the message, mutters an oath and an unquotable remark about the girth of lower bodily parts of the Secretary, and says, "All right, son, you'll have to do as a substitute. The rest of the cabinet and a few of the diplomatic corps are setting off this morning afoot on my new exercise hike. We're going from here over through Rock Creek Park. I want you to mark my route with those 1st Calvary guidons from my old outfit that your blimpy boss sent along with you."

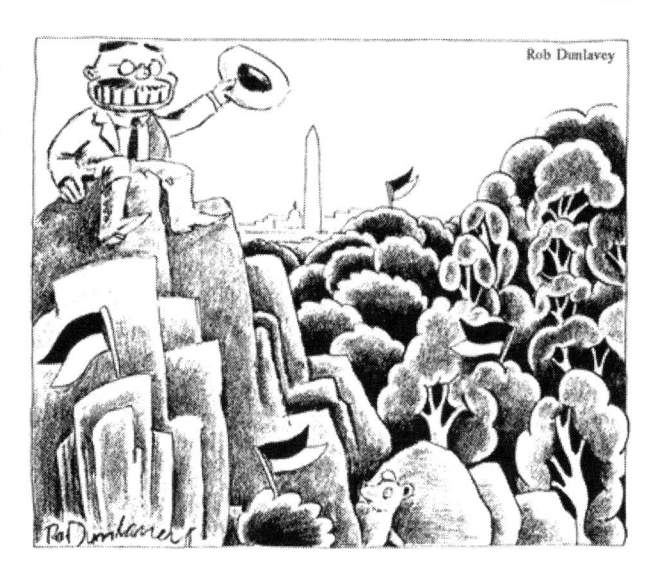

They move to the foyer, and the President hefts one and says, "Ah, ha! Bully! We should have had these going up Kettle Hill! They're just right for visibility, with both red and white to show in the woods. You can drive the standards into the ground as we go, so stragglers can find their way on our azimuth. I always go just one bearing, you see, and we don't stop regardless of obstacles."

Shortly thereafter that morning, the aide found himself huffing and puffing up a steep incline and up rock faces, with pants dripping from the last creek crossing, while the President charged ahead. He planted the last cavalry flag, then looked back to see the entourage stumbling along trying to keep up. He noted that the Swedish ambassador, curiously, was making some kind of notes in his field book, and was surprised to see a sketch of the Army flag on a page as his excellency caught up and passed him.

Another cabinet officer, Mr. Elihu Root, later vaguely reminisced that the President often announced his intended westerly course at the outset–shouting, "Let's head for the Orient. Bully!" Mr. Root was pleased to turn over his duties to Mr. Taft and be done with all that damn "orienting".

It may be only a coincidence that the very next year our youngest President was the first American to receive the Nobel Prize, but it may not be a fluke that that same young aide was soon posted to Sweden and the cavalry flags vanished from the front hall closet of 1600 Pennsylvania Avenue.

Yes, dear reader—that same man responsible for a great number of the US national parks and forests, the Rough Rider, namesake of the "Teddy Bear", and endorser of "the strenuous life"—he must have started it all! Thanks, T.R.!!!

[Editor's note: Like most Orienteering maps, the above article is based on careful research and field work, and is about 95% accurate, the other most critical 5% being pure conjecture!]

Published in *Orienteering North America* November 1988 issue.

THE PONTIUS ARROWHEAD

Decades from now, as our children's children ponder over the arcane history and lore of their ancestors' rudimentary attempts at Orienteering, questions may arise over the origin of the lonely little mark stuck by itself down at the south end of O' maps. Well, for those future researchers who locate this hallowed publication, here is the story. It seems that one Ron P., a famous and very fast M21 elite type, a member of the notorious Blue Star Komplex (BSK) and while affiliated with the Nisqually O' Club of Olympia/Tacoma, once ran a championship relay at the equally infamous Forest of Nisene Marks venue in California. At an early control, his compass and folded map somehow slipped in his hand, and when he reset them for his next leg, a ghastly 180° error developed! By the time he caught it, all hope for his relay team winning had been wiped out!!

All for the lack of a visible arrowhead? Yes, it's true! If this could have happened to an Elite, imagine what the rest of the world's orienteers were doing, after folding up those big maps to manageable size or to grasp neatly with a thumb compass on top! The magnetic north lines are usually carefully drawn spaced across the map, and names are right-side up for "North-Up", but those arrowheads and lettering often disappear from sight as maps are turned and folded. Thus North becomes South, but only at the most inopportune time! (Murphy never heard of this one!)

Some astute orienteers had for some time been placing supplemental arrowheads here and there on their maps during events, but it occurred to this author, hearing Ron's sad story while making my first map, that a little arrowhead or two belonged down at the South end of those lines, at some likely spot(s) which would remain visible if the entire North end of the map got turned under.

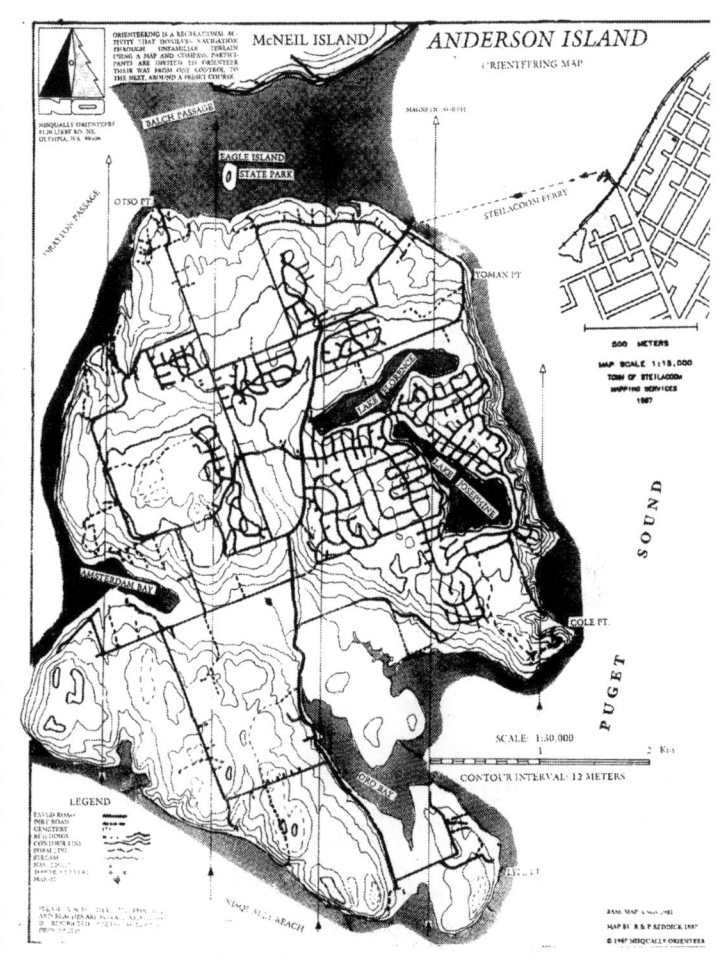

Well, the rest is history! Sure enough, other Northwest U.S. mapmakers adopted this simple convention, and little-by-little the thing spread, and the Pontius name stuck! Eventually it finally won IOF approval (after several decades). No one ever heard of Ron again, but his namesake THE PONTIUS ARROWHEAD has made him immortal!

Ron Pontius now lives in North Carolina, and was just married to Chae-Im Santos.

Published in *Orienteering North America* June 1989 issue.

ORIENTEERS NEED WATER—SERIOUSLY
A Competitor's, Meet Director's, and Course-Setter's Guide

Water, Water, Everywhere

Water, water, everywhere (in your shoes, on your glasses, down your back in the northwest region, during half of our 12-month season of Orienteering)—BUT NOT A DROP TO DRINK! Why? No water points, unfindable ones, or dry ones, in meets ranging from local meets to some large A-meets. Yet, the body is fueled by water, is about 90% water, and just won't function correctly without it. With insufficient water, excessive body temperature can occur, possibly heat exhaustion or heat stroke, certainly fatigue and lower work efficiency, and perhaps an increased risk of accidents and injury. Even the most well-conditioned and trained athletes must take on sufficient liquids for best performance, and the rest of us amateur orienteers must try to maintain the right level of "liquidity" to do our best.

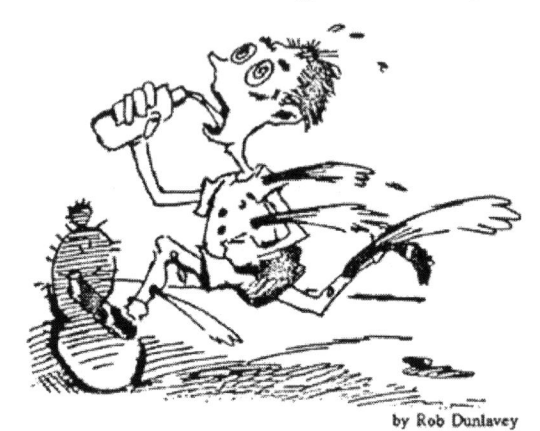

How Much?

So what are the right amounts to take, when, and how often? The doctors and other medical practitioners I've asked usually have only a rough idea of the needs of athletes, but much research has been done by sports medicine specialists and companies that manufacture sports drinks. These experts offer the following guidelines:

Competitor's Drinking Plan

2 hours before event/workout: 32 oz. or .95 liters, drink slowly!
15 minutes before start: 15 oz.
Each 15-30 min. during run: 8-10 oz.
After finish: 32 oz.

Note that this is fluid intake—cold water is best, cheapest, and for dieters, has zero calories; sports drinks* or orange juice are also good if diluted to 1/2 or 1/4 strength, to allow quick processing by the stomach. Needless to say, sugary drinks and alcoholic ones are out, until the event is over!

Plan Your Drinking

The orienteer must plan ahead to meet these fluid requirements, keeping in mind that the feeling of thirst comes way too late to be a good indicator of fluid need. The before and after event drinking are mostly the individual's responsibility to supply, although most good meet organizers will provide adequate water at both the Start and the Finish areas, and at any warm-up area. Those organizers will hopefully provide unlocked facilities or dense forest for relieving the kidneys just before the start, also.

by Rob Dunlavey

Published in *Orienteering North America* July 1989 issue.

On the course, the competitor must first identify the marked locations of water controls, which hopefully are right at the regular course control features. If any water points should be elsewhere, (not recommended, since that becomes another "control" to find), determine at the outset how to reach them in selecting your route. Then the orienteer must remember to stop and drink the full 8-10 oz., even if only little 3 oz. cups are there. The first water stop is probably the most important, even though you have absolutely no thirst, the weather is cool, and you think you're doing great! By the second water point on a long course, you could be seriously dehydrated, not thinking clearly, and only just starting to feel a thirst, and the water consumed there may not have much chance to be digested before you finish. And some of us never know for sure when we'll reach that Finish area!

Officials, Take Notice!

For the meet directors and course setters, plus the vetters who inspect the courses just before the first competitors start, here's a planning table to copy and keep handy for planning and checking. It is based on US and Canadian Orienteering rules and guidelines on course refreshments, which require water at least every 2.5 to 3 km. of actual travel (not beeline), with 8 oz. (.25 liters) for each visitor there:

Orienteering Water Table

Water Required for each 10 Competitors (in gallons)

Course	Typical Length	Start	On Course Distance 1/3	1/2	2/3	Finish	Total
1 or White	2.3km	1.2	-	-	-	2.5	3.7
2 Yellow	3.0	1.2	-	0.8	-	2.5	4.5
3 Orange	4.0	1.2	-	0.8	-	2.5	4.5
4 Green	4.5	1.2	-	0.8	-	2.5	4.5
5 Red	5.5	1.2	0.8	-	0.8	2.5	5.3
6 Blue	6.5	1.2	0.8	-	0.8	2.5	5.3
7 Elite	7.5	1.2	0.8	(0.8)	0.8	2.5	5.3
				hot?			(6.1)
8 Elite	10.0	1.2	0.8	0.8	0.8	2.5	6.1

For example, to use this table to find your water needs for a local event, with courses 1 through 4 offered to 40 people, evenly divided, and no common water points, you'll need a total of 3.7 + 4.5 + 4.5 + 4.5 gal = 17.2 gal total, to be placed at the Start (5 ea. 1-gal containers), the Finish (4 ea. 2 1/2 gal containers or equivalent), and at three controls near the midpoint of courses 2, 3, and 4 (0.8 gal each). Course 1 (White) normally would not need a water control, but remember that these are minimums, and hot and/or windy weather plus difficult navigation should impel you to provide additional stops.

One Last Observation

One last observation–some course setters love to place the water jugs and cups some distance away from the control shown on the control card (the cup symbol). It is usually argued that to prevent lingering orienteers from giving the control away, the water point must be away from the control. But why not just deliberately make the point an easy-to-find control, or use a place where people drinking are not easily seen? The essence of Orienteering is not the finding of the control itself anyway, but the route choice and successful navigation of the leg enroute!

See Nancy Clark's article "Is Water Best?" In the May 1987 *ONA*.

[Ed. note: Remember, this article represents Bob Reddick's opinion. If you have questions about his advice, consult your physician or your local Water Department.]

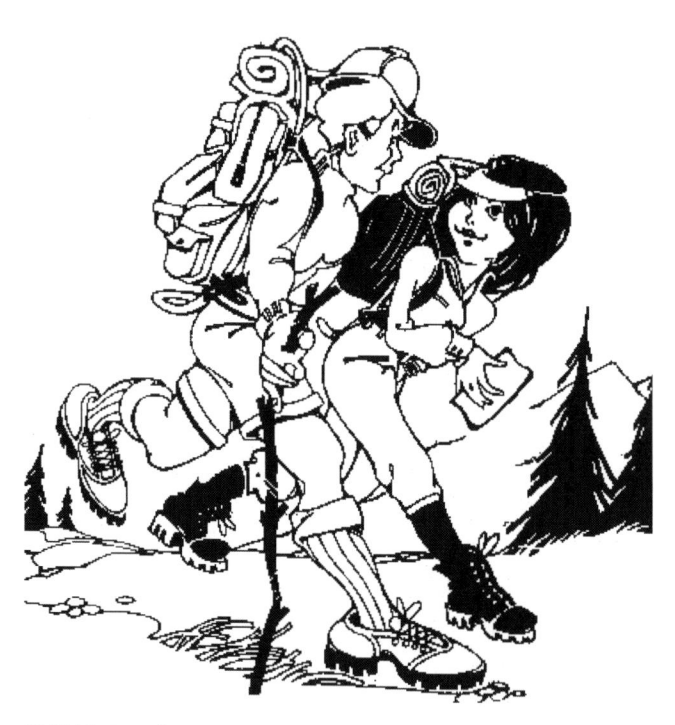

"I did bring the wine, Neil. Oh, do you think Bob's 10-lb. pack rule is just a joke?"

"Yep, Gail. And speaking of jokes, I snuck Rod's ice bag of Foster's out of his pack and replaced it with six big rocks!"

BOOK REVIEWS – Three Navigation Books

Land Navigation Handbook

The Sierra Club Guide to Map and Compass by W. S. Kals, Sierra Club Books, San Francisco, ©1983

The first half of this book is devoted to an excellent discussion of maps and compasses; how to purchase, use, and carry them. The black-and-white illustrations are frequent and helpful. Chapters 8 through 12 cover magnetic declination, use of altimeters, and obtaining directions from the sky, which are of only minor interest to orienteers. The most useful tip is well-covered: marking your USGS or other non-Orienteering map with magnetic north lines in advance of any hike, to save the nuisance of adjusting for declination.

The last chapter captures a lot of the important tricks and strategies of cross-country navigation, including the regular use at appropriate times of thumbing the map, pace-counting, time estimation and creative route-planning. The making and use of pace-counting gauges to stick on your compass is discussed in some detail. For example, if your personalized pace-counting ruler used on the next leg shows a distance of 400 paces, but you're going through the woods without a trail, you'll know that it will be 600 paces before you will see the control. (You might even put your non-level pacing factor numbers on such scales, perhaps color-coded.) A good index and a sample 5-color topographic map are included.

This book is recommended for the frequent hiker, canoeist, or other outdoors person who frequently uses maps.

Be Expert with Map and Compass

The Orienteering Handbook by Bjorn Kjellstrom, Charles Scribner's Sons, N.Y., ©1976

The standard handbook for orienteers, written by the former Swedish champion and one of the founders of U.S. Orienteering, this is designed for beginners, scout groups, newcomers to map and compass work, and outdoors people in general. It covers the basics in types of Orienteering courses and how to plan and organize simple meets. Materials included are a practice compass, protractor, and a sample of an orienteering map. Illustrations and figures arc frequent and designed for the beginner. Tests are included for review of principles discussed.

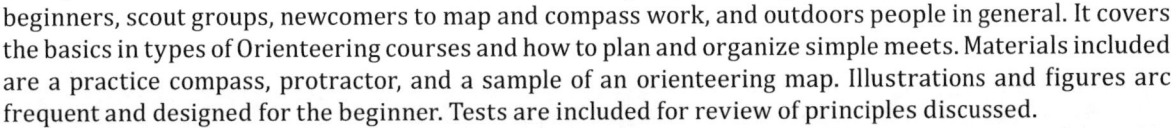

The sections on map-reading and compass use are excellent, and the user should have no trouble trying out the information in the field. The book strongly emphasizes that skills must be developed by actual practice on many occasions in the field. The Postmortem is briefly discussed, where perhaps some of the best learning takes place. That's when immediately after finishing your course, you mingle with others and pick up experiences, tips and ideas on what others did, such as better or worse routes, different attack points, and useful navigational techniques. I have found that the fastest person on my course usually provides the best information.

This is the ideal first reference book for any new orienteer, and would make a good gift for juniors getting into their first navigational experiences.

Published in *Orienteering North America* November 1989 issue.

Cross-Country Navigation

Outdoor Recreation in Australia by Rod Phillips, Neil Phillips and Graham Foley, Perth, ©1989

The new book by three "Aussie" rogaining champions is the result of an attempted update of the standard and only text on the sport of rogaining, the 24 hour cross-country score-Orienteering events that originated in Australia. They got carried away with their update and have produced an expanded, very thorough and readable cross-country navigation text which covers map-reading skills and compass use, as well as the use of celestial navigation, and the inclusion of tests of materials covered. Color photos and illustrations brighten the work; and case histories of navigation in competitions and life-threatening situations keep the reader turning pages.

For the rogaine competitor, the book is most useful in planning, training with your partner, and equipping yourself for this mini-adventure. For the rogaine event organizer, the book is a must. Tips are offered on course planning, safety, and catering (the food service is absolutely critical to a successful event, based on the reviewer's experiences as both a competitor and an organizer of rogaines). Appendices cover most everything needed for organizing and running a rogaine, and an equipment checklist for competitors is included. The use of down-under terms such as "bushwalker," "torch" and "paddock" add interest for the North American reader, and the section on the history of rogaining leads up to the spread of the sport internationally with the recent forming of the International Rogaining Federation.

An important point is made by the authors on remaining independent, both a rule and a part of the spirit of both orienteering and rogaining. I've often been led astray or mistakenly revised my perfect control attack plan by other competitors in the vicinity when I assumed they knew what they were doing, or knew more than I did. The example in the book describes one rogaine team deliberately following another at night, expecting to be led right to the control. The leaders dropped quietly into the bracken and removed their "guiding light," which left the followers to quickly consult their maps, to decide on their likely whereabouts, and then to confidently strike off in a direction that took them off the map!

This book is obviously my favorite, not just for the rogaining, but for the wealth of useful cross-country techniques applicable to most Orienteering courses.

The first two books are available through bookstores, or Orienteering equipment suppliers; the Australian book is being distributed in North America by the Washington State Orienteering Association, PO Box 111977, Tacoma, WA 98413-1977.

Land Navigation Handbook and *Be Expert with Map and Compass* were updated in 2005 and 2009, respectively, and are available on Amazon.com. *Cross-Country Navigation* is planned for an update soon.

ARE YOU READY FOR WHITE?
Ideas for the Competitor and the Designer

What can the beginning orienteer expect in encountering the first map course? What should a boy or girl aged 12 or under expect in a championship meet course? How about the men and women of any age who prefer to do only the 1.5 to 3 km easy map walk, without the need to plow through off-trail brush or forest? In every Orienteering meet, from the local ones to the big championships, there is a course designed for all of these enthusiasts, called the WHITE COURSE.

Tough Puzzle for Beginners?

Sometimes event organizers don't have enough time or resources to provide much training or an escorted newcomer's introduction to this multifaceted sport. So a newcomer may be given a map and punch card, directed from the registration to the starting position, and there given a start time and a "Go!" You're then on your own to navigate the course to the finish, punching in at controls in order per the description sheet, which lists the control codes and describes the features to be found.

For planning purposes, about 10% of all entrants at a large 'A' meet compete on the White Course, and all newcomers at local meets do this course. These competitors are the future of Orienteering, and must not be disappointed in the quality and suitability of the courses they encounter!

White courses must be very carefully designed to fit the needs and abilities of these young and/or inexperienced people; too often, the course designers overdesign them. As the IOF points out, "it is very easy to make these courses too difficult. The course planner should be careful not to estimate the difficulty based on his walking speed, when surveying the area." Sometimes designers forget just how challenging it is to set off in a new area and try to read the special Orienteering map, while working against a clock. Any trail junction becomes a puzzle, and some maps are very hard to even read, much less understand. So for the first-time orienteer, simplicity is the goal, and it can never be too simple! The novice must finish, and with a feeling of successfully accomplishing something. The more experienced White course entrant will be going for better speed, and outdoing other competitors.

A White Course Critique

Let's walk you through the White Course set at the U.S. Championships at Annadel State Park, California, in 1989. The idea here is to see how each leg, from control to control, might be done, what changes or improvements could be made in course setting, and what the orienteer should be looking for in doing the course. If you have the November issue of this magazine, you have the inserted map of the course. This course is shown on the description sheet as 2.6 km long, with 90 meters of climb and 6 controls.

The Start triangle is about a 15-minute walk, 900 meters uphill from the parking along Channel Drive. The location shows a lot of yellow, or open land around, with some black dots representing boulders. Control #1 is shown as a trail junction (dashed lines joining) 160 m. straight ahead (south) from the Start. So we just walk ahead fast through the open area, to near where the white (forest) shows on the map, looking for a trail to join ours from the right. The control should be right there. On this White course, the flag should be hung just beyond the junction, in plain sight, just to the left down the trail. This gets the beginner started the right direction for the next leg. The map circle is centered just before the junction—not good.

Control #2 is about 450 meters and 7 contour lines (brown squiggles marking 5 meter changes in elevation) up and around the left of the big green-shaded hill on the good trail to the first tiny yellow spot

Published in *Orienteering North America* January 1990 issue.

(a clearing). This leg should be a cinch, since the flag should be found right along the trail in plain sight. Just to be sure that you don't stop too soon in some open area too small to map, or the woods are so pretty you forget to look for the control until you've gone too far, you could try estimating the distance, either by pacing it off at maybe 70 paces for each 100 meters (or your factor), and/or maybe timing it at 1 minute for each 100 meters walking (again, use your own experience factor). Another way is to watch for all those tiny dots on the map (rocky ground) to show up along the trail, then go about 100 meters further. This leg should lake less than 5 minutes. Remember to punch in at each control!

Too Hard for Beginners?

Control #3 is very hard—first forward on the trail 80 m. to a junction with a very faint and hard-to-read trail going to the right–then on for about 400 meters to another faint trail junction, then left to where the forest (white color) hits the clearing (yellow). [Note: These two junctions, the very faint trail, and the route choice decisions should not be a part of this course.] Another way there is to go along the main trail from #2 to the huge clearing, until the 3 side trails to your left are passed, and #4 can be spotted at the green spot (heavy vegetation) to your right—then go from #4 just 150 meters uphill through the woods to the next clearing, and look for the control just as you get to the small trail. This would normally require the use of a compass for accuracy, for it's easy to lose track of a straight line route while going uphill through the trees.

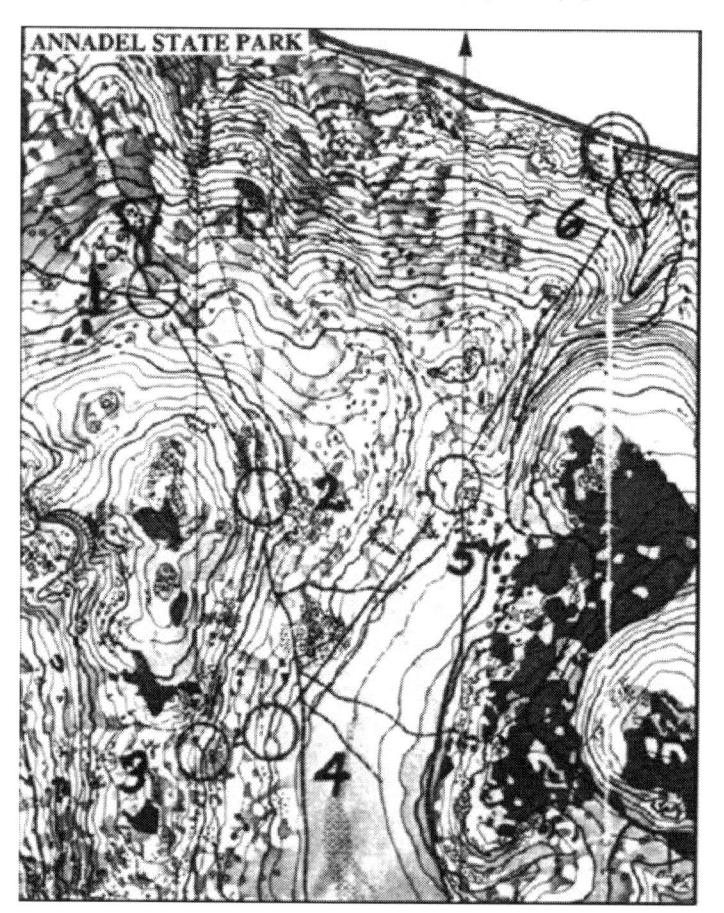

There were also two other controls on other courses nearby, which could confuse you. Be sure to match the control code shown on the description sheet before punching. This is also where it would be nice to find water on a hot day. This could have been a common control for the White, Orange, and even Red courses, with water for all.

Hansel & Gretel Technique!

Assuming you've found #3, you get to #4 by heading roughly east to the huge clearing, then searching along its western edge for the heavy vegetation at the edge of the woods. No handrails here! *[Ed. note: ONA believes that there should have been streamers as a guide to the clearing.]* Of course, if you just came back from #4 to find #3, you'll look for the footprints or bread-crumbs you left enroute, or better—the little details you memorized as you went. (Those other orienteers may also be wearing size 5 ½ Nikes and be using whole wheat, too!) If you're really lost (whoops, orienteers never get lost—we just have to relocate sometimes), you may wish to find the main trail again and retreat along it back to #2. Then start off again, this time pace-counting and timing yourself, while carefully checking off everything shown on the map, and trying to watch the uphill and downhill parts, and even the little wiggles in the trail.

Many orienteers have found that going quickly back to the last control or major feature they passed where they can find themselves again exactly on the map is the fastest way to recover—it's called "bailing out", and many advanced orienteers do this within the FIRST MINUTE after the control doesn't show up at the "right" location. There are single trees, boulders, and many vegetation boundaries around #3 and #4 that might be used by an advanced orienteer for navigation, but watch out, it's easy to get unmapped things to match up in your mind with what you see on the map. *[Ed note: We call this "mental earth-moving".]*

Now you're finally headed for #5, in an intermittent creek bed (blue dashed line) near a trail bend. So you head northeast 550 meters across the edge of the big clearing, along the fainter trail, to the bigger trail and then to the woods edge. You can see on the map to go about 50 meters into the woods to the north, with a creek bed to your left. You watch carefully to make sure you're on the right trail, for there are unmapped trails around, and that you see the creek and don't go too far. Remember not to expect to see water in the creek bed in the middle of a hot, dry summer. The climb down to the creek bed was rocky with dangerous footing, so the control should have properly been located just off the trail.

After punching in at #5, you keep on the trail curling to the right (east) for 120 meters until it joins the main trail heading downhill to the finish area. At the junction, the course setter should have placed another control to be sure to turn you the correct direction, for this is another route choice decision. Look carefully at the map, and you'll see that a right turn here would take you back to the big clearing or uphill through heavy forest, instead of down the steep hillside the way you should go. After going about 550 meters another route choice comes up—straight north on a narrower trail, or looping back left on the S-shaped main trail to #6. Either way gets you there, but the north route looks shorter and faster. But in some conditions the main S-trail could be faster, by being clear of deadfall, loose rock, or mud, with an easy crossing of the creek, while that shortcut route could be nasty and difficult. This is part of the challenge and fun in advanced Orienteering to have to make these route choice decisions for routes and maps you've never been on before!

After you punch at #6, the 80 meters down to the double-circle symbol finish line is usually flagged, and the description sheet will tell you this. Be sure to check it, for the flagging (used-car lot bunting or engineer tape) really helps to get you home, and it often can be seen from a distance to clue you in where that #6 is, too!

Well, you've traveled about 3130 meters on this 2.6 km course, counting the dog-leg from 4 to 3 and back to 4, made several route choices, needed the compass once or twice, and saw a good variety of vegetation and terrain. At a fast walk, with lots of map-reading and no serious mistakes, you probably did it in 39 minutes. During the actual meet, it was reported that Dennis Steinemann of Switzerland ran this course in 19:03 (M12A) and Bent Buraas from Norway (now BAOC) did it in 35:17, so the length was OK.

White Course Guidelines

As a summary of the International O-Federation Guidelines to Course Planning, the US O-Federation binder, and Canadian O-Federation A-Meet Organizing Manual, you should expect that:

The course should be of a length that no one can finish in under 25 minutes, but that any beginner on the first solo outing can finish. The Canadian guideline is 1.5 to 2.5 km in length, but the 25 minute finish time for the winner is more important. Anything shorter than this is not enough challenge or activity for someone who may have traveled a long distance to get to the event.

Most all legs should be along "handrails", like a trail, road, stone wall, fence, lake shore, etc., and maybe streamers on a leg through woods if absolutely necessary to insure a good handrail. In this respect, the White Course is very much like a string course with no string, but with a highly visible and easy to follow mapped "string" always in sight of the competitor. Avoid very hilly, wet, or marshy areas, and wild or rough forest. Developed areas are necessary for sufficient handrails. Avoid hard-to-read areas on the map. Only one, repeat, ONE route choice is to be likely between controls. The legs should not cross each other.

It's strongly advised not to separate the starts for the lower and higher level courses—development and the future life of this sport needs the mix and interaction of all levels of competitors. The common start area may be somewhat limiting for the course designers, but for the good of the sport ways should be found to find the single point where all courses can begin.

Short legs and interesting, varying features are desired, and you should expect legs of 150 to 300 meters, rarely longer. The features selected, such as large boulders, cliffs, stream junctions, or single trees must be easily visible from the trail or other handrail, even by the shortest competitor. No nearby similar features must be there for confusion. If the control is used for other courses, keep it as a beginner's control. No compass work is to be required on White, and no need for reading of contour lines!

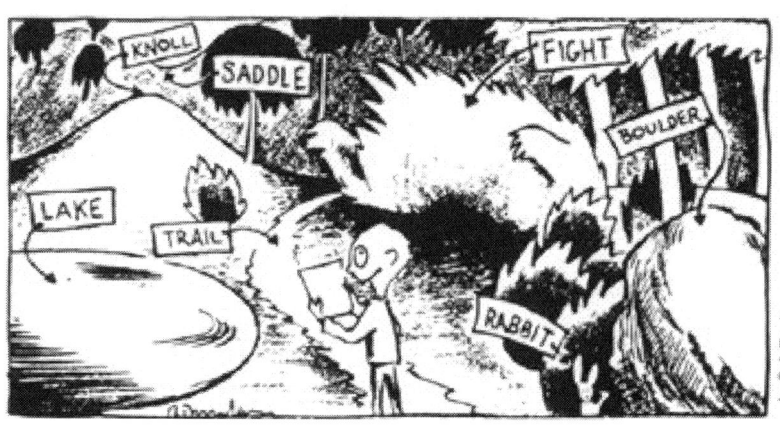

The control marker should be easily seen from a distance, and not hidden behind the feature! It also must be easily visible from any direction, and particularly from the handrail. If it is at a trail junction, it should be placed a short distance down the trail heading toward the next control, so no route choice error is likely. Where the course may allow a person to choose to leave the handrail and take a shortcut through woods or rough terrain, there must be no danger of getting lost or injured on that route.

The course should be tested by a skilled orienteer to see that the above objectives are met, that the time at a slow jog or fast walk is at least 25 minutes, and that no other control markers of other courses might be visible to confuse the White runners.

If the map and event area have been used in previous events, check the results and old description sheets to make the new course different and to adjust for correct time, length, and for variety in features for controls.

Make sure that there is sufficient water at both the start and the finish, and on a warm or sunny day place water at the midpoint control for the wayfarer orienteers. Remind White course entrants to "tank up" before starting out, and to return to the finish or go to the safety direction if lost or confused. Also remind everyone of the time limit (usually 3 hours) and the course closure time.

Everyone on the White Course!

At local events and non-championship competitions, the White course is an ideal warm-up jog for higher-level course participants. It gives you the chance to get the blood flowing and body loosened up, the mind active in matching map to terrain, and even compass practice. Or why not walk a beginner or family around the course, answering questions and pointing out potential errors, while secretly looking for your own optimum route? Finished your tougher course and still have energy to burn? Get together an impromptu Sprint-O on the White Course (wait till the beginners are done, or they'll get spooked by the heavy-breathing hotshots hovering over them at the punches!)

A Designer's Challenge

Remember, everyone is a winner on the White Course, and the White Course is for everyone. Designers are challenged to make then as perfect as they try to do for the Blue and Red courses, so the White runner can expect a quality and interesting experience at every event. Designers should ask a vetter to slowly jog the course after the flags or controls are placed, to check on all the guidelines listed above.

And beginners—after a few events, if you see your name at the top of every White course result list, everyone will tell you "it's time to move up to Yellow"!

So—ARE YOU READY FOR WHITE?

ORIENTEERING WORD PUZZLE

Y	R	O	C	K	F	I	E	L	D	E	C	L	I	N	A	T	I	O	N
E	A	T	T	A	C	K	P	O	I	N	T	E	L	O	R	T	N	O	C
L	C	V	E	C	I	R	T	E	M	M	A	R	G	O	T	O	H	P	Q
L	O	V	E	G	E	T	A	T	I	O	N	B	O	U	N	D	A	R	Y
O	M	S	H	T	R	O	N	C	I	T	E	N	G	A	M	K	F	N	D
W	A	C	S	G	F	O	R	E	S	T	A	R	T	E	E	Y	I	N	N
C	P	A	N	G	O	O	K	I	N	A	I	D	H	E	D	G	E	I	S
O	M	L	O	N	G	O	R	E	E	N	T	R	A	N	T	G	U	U	A
U	A	E	I	T	E	R	R	A	I	N	O	I	S	S	E	R	P	E	D
R	W	A	T	E	R	P	O	I	N	T	T	H	T	L	N	O	S	E	D
S	S	A	P	M	O	C	B	M	U	H	T	E	R	U	P	S	T	I	L
E	H	P	I	C	A	T	C	H	I	N	G	F	E	A	T	U	R	E	E
K	I	O	R	O	O	T	S	T	O	C	K	S	T	R	O	I	E	J	I
A	U	N	C	L	I	M	B	A	B	L	E	H	T	R	I	T	A	U	G
L	L	D	S	E	L	T	T	E	N	T	E	H	V	B	A	N	M	N	G
B	L	U	E	C	O	U	R	S	E	N	I	A	G	O	R	I	G	C	A
A	A	E	D	I	R	E	S	P	O	C	O	M	P	A	S	S	L	T	B
I	W	C	A	N	O	E	O	S	K	T	F	F	O	G	N	I	M	I	A
R	I	V	E	R	U	T	A	E	F	G	N	I	T	C	E	L	L	O	C
G	E	T	A	G	A	I	T	E	R	S	C	O	R	E	O	A	D	N	S

AIMINGOFF
ATTACKPOINT
BAGGIE
BLUECOURSE
CANOEO
CATCHINGFEATURE
COLLECTINGFEATURE
COMPASS
CONTROL
COPSE
DECLINATION
DEPRESSION
DESCRIPTION
DNF
DNS

FOREST
GAITERS
GOOKINAID
HEDGE
JUNCTION
KNOLL
LAKE
LEGEND
LONGO
MAGNETICNORTH
MAP
NETTLES
ORIENTEERING
OSUIT

OVT
PATH
PHOTOGRAMMETRIC
POND
REENTRANT
RIDE
RIVER
ROCKFIELD
ROGAINE
ROOTSTOCK
ROUTE
RUIN
SADDLE
SCALE

SCOREO
SPUR
START
STREAM
SWAMP
TERRAIN
THICKET
THUMBCOMPASS
TRAIL
UNCLIMBABLE
VEGETATIONBOUNDARY
WALL
WATERPOINT
YELLOWCOURSE

Published in *Orienteering North America* January and August 1990 issues.

O-ATLAS – Washington State and Puget Sound

This is a continuation of the O-atlas series begun back in August 1986 with the St. Louis area.

For Orienteering travelers and those who might want to explore some new terrain while on business, sightseeing, or vacation in the Puget Sound area of Washington, here are the available maps which will allow you to practice your navigation skills or just enjoy some nice walks in beautiful surroundings.

For those coming to the two-week Asia-Pacific Orienteering Celebration in August 1990, these maps will help you get acquainted with the terrain and mapping conventions here. For information on local meets not published in this magazine, you may call the COC Orienteering Hotline at (206)783-3866 any time.

All maps are 5-color IOF standard, scales 1:5000 to 1:15000, with contour interval usually 3 meters, unless otherwise noted.

All of these maps can be ordered from the Washington State Orienteering Association, P.O. Box 411977, Tacoma, WA 98411; most of them can also be purchased at the local Recreation Equipment Inc. (REI) stores.

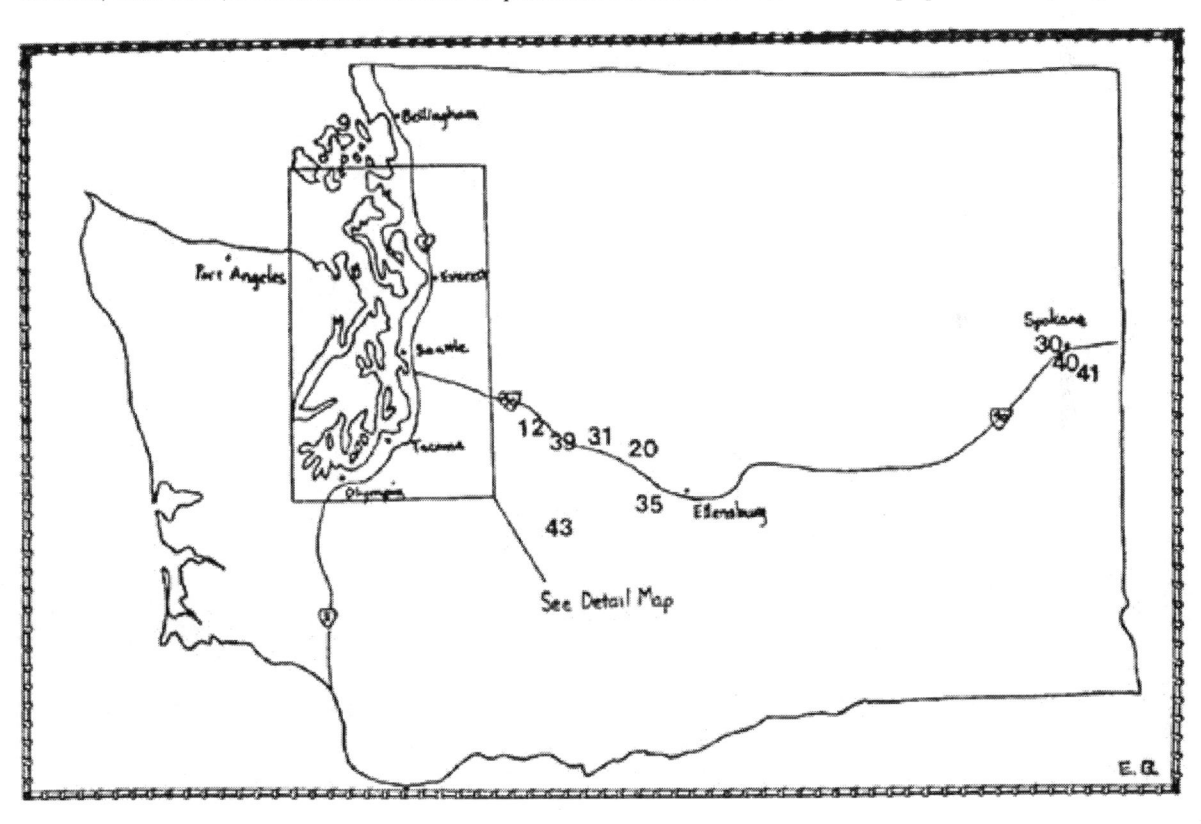

#	Name
1.	Discovery Park
2.	Drunken Charlie Lake
3.	Lk Sammamish State Park
4.	Lake Tradition
5.	Lincoln Park
6.	Luther Burbank Park
7.	Lynndale Park
8.	Marymoor Park
9.	Moran State Park
10.	Seward Park
11.	St Edward State Park
12.	Trollhaugen
13.	Union Bay
14.	Woodland Park
15.	Ft. Casey
16.	Point Defiance Park
17.	Wright Park
18.	Ft. Steilacoom County Park
19.	Spanaway Park North
20.	Cle Elum Ridge
21.	Tenalquot
22.	Bridle Trails State Park
23.	Pioneer/Island Crest Park
24.	Priest Point Park (B&W, 1:7500,5)
25.	Hamlin Park (B&W,1:7500,3)
26.	Evergreen State College (B&W,1:5000,3)
27.	Anderson Island (B&W,1:30000,12)
28.	NAD Park, Bangor
29.	St. Martin's Campus (1:5000,3)
30.	Riverside Park, Spokane
31.	APOC'90 & World Cup venue
32.	Univ of Washington Campus
33.	Kelsey Creek Park
34.	Magnuson Park
35.	Old Durr Road
36.	Farrel-McWhirter
37.	Forest Park (B&W, 1:5000)
38.	Ballard (bicycle)
39.	Easton Grade
40.	Lincoln (Spokane) (B&W, 1:5000)
41.	Manito Park (Spokane)
42.	Robinswood (1:3000)
43.	Tumac Mountain (B&W, 1:32000,40m)
44.	Vashon Island
45.	Volunteer Park (B&W, 1:3000)
46.	Yelm High School (B&W, 1:3000)

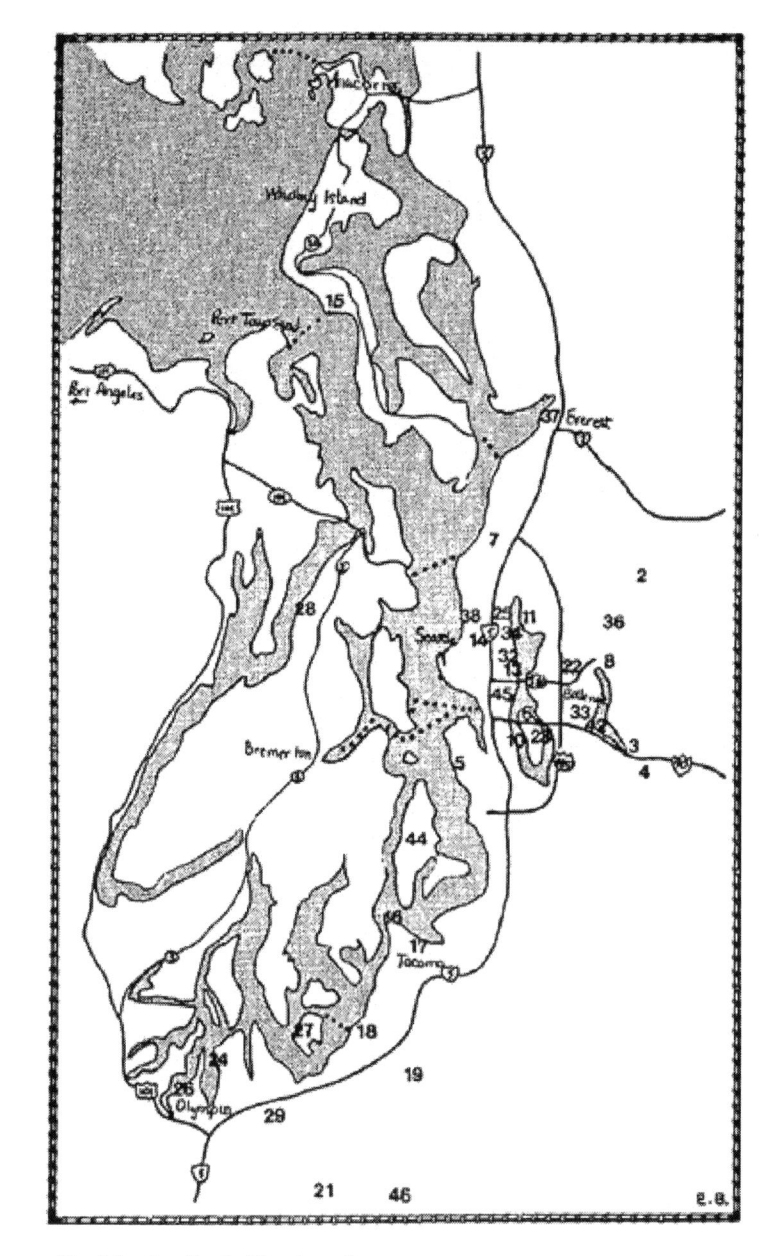

A CANOE O'

One memorable misadventure happened in the summer of 1992, at the University of Washington campus and Portage Bay: a Canoe Orienteering event. Pat, a new-to-orienteering guy, and I were halfway through our course, having done the controls on Marsh and Foster Islands. We watched with astonishment as an up-side-down canoe was rapidly moving across the island on four running legs! It was an extremely creative portage, but not against the rules. We did one control on shore near the Montlake Bridge, where Pat slipped in the mud, getting wet shoes and pant legs.

We then paddled back across the busy power-boat passage and past the old shellhouse (used as a seaplane hanger in WWI) and the rental boats and dock. Near the new Conibear shellhouse, we found the next control marker tied up high upon a tree at the water's edge. I got out of the canoe and climbed up onto a large branch of the tree, and then paused to consider our next moves.

I instructed Pat and our teammate to paddle back to the dock, while I got this control, and would then cut through the brush, run along the service road east of the football stadium to get our last control near the old shellhouse, then rejoin them at the Finish. No sooner had they moved beyond hearing range, the branch I was standing on broke (it turned out to be rotten), dropping me three feet and scattering my glasses, compass and map. After recovering with much difficulty and punching the control, I discovered the brush I had to pass through next were ten-foot tall Blackberry bushes with thorns, which looked impassable. I considered swimming or wading through the lily-pad covered water, or trying to bash my way through the blackberry bushes, using the big broken tree limb. I tried that for about two minutes with the blackberry bush fiercely resisting. Sitting down, feeling trapped and frustrated, I saw the solution! It was passable by merely crawling beneath the bushes, which worked with surprisingly few minor scratches.

I ran to the last control, and then on to meet my team at the dock, ready to apologize for being several minutes delayed. However, there was no canoe or team! Where were they? Then I spotted them further down the dock area, emptying water out of our canoe. Pat said that a distant speedboat caused a wake that caught them off-guard and caused the boat to capsize. Several orienteers in a passing canoe must have been in a hurry, as they made no effort to stop to see if Pat and our teammate could swim or required assistance. Our teammate lost his glasses. [Note: We never saw him again at any other event.] Although somewhat soggy, wet and scratched up, we triumphantly finished the event! Yea!

Over many Canoe-O' events, this turned out to be the most memorable!

A CHANGE IN COMPETITIVE STYLE

How the "Damn the torpedoes, full speed ahead!" Technique became the "I'm sick, so I'll just try to survive this course!" Technique.

I realize that some of you gentle readers have already been bored to tears with the first part of this tale, since the 1989 Washington State Centennial Games in Spokane. However, the second part from the September 1992 Washington State Championships held in Cle Elum Ridge hosted by Cascade, with cookie support by Ellensburg OC, is brand new.

First, a little background on me, I am a M55A class and have been in orienteering for two years. I attempted my previously used style on orienteering courses, including the first day on the new Riverside Park map. This map was new for the first Summer Games and the 1989 Washington Centennial. Al Smith of SLOC and Ulf Koster of Germany did the field work with R.D. and Gary McCausland and Pat Albright getting it in final form. My mode had always been to go at a fairly fast pace at first and then speed up whenever things looked right or runnable trails looked useful. I use the backward planning technique of CARTT or Control, Attack point, Route, Terrain, and Tempo (or time) to select my whole route from control to control. But in practice, I'd always take the somewhat aggressive and risky routes which, while very direct, involved all the navigational difficulties the clever course designer had devised to challenge the competitors. This usually led to very good results on say nine controls on a 10-control Green course. And to a loss of about 30 minutes on just one control which often was the easiest-looking one. (I sense the reader's head nodding in recognition of a common foible in us all.)

I also previously quickly considered, but just as quickly discarded, the looping, long-way-around routes as not too much fun or challenging—such as coming in the back way to the feature to see the control bag early after taking the longer way there. This method if used takes advantage of the elephant tracks and sometimes an orienteer departing that control for the next one.

For this Spokane event, my wife Pat and I had driven 6 hours overnight from Steilacoom on Puget Sound after flying in from California, sleeping an hour in the car, then competing in the hot weather of Day One. My result the first day was dismal—although I made only one navigational mistake in mid-course when I tried to remove a nylon long-sleeved O' shirt to cool off while running. I got it tangled in my compass cord tied to my wrist, and wandered far enough off my track to make a parallel error costing 5 minutes relocation time. I ended up dead last among the men (all classes) in the event, so knew where I'd start the next day in the Chase Start planned. (Chase Start: competitors start spaced out in order of finish times from first day—so if you pass someone, you've gained a place, etc.)

Pat and I spent the afternoon taking in other Centennial Games events, and were most humbled about our personal athletic endeavors while watching the top competitors vying in Wheelchair Tennis! On Sunday, both of us were feeling bad, and just 15 minutes before my dead-last start time I felt the urgent need to visit the outhouse, and didn't quite make it there before a sudden diarrhea attack occurred. I just had time to change my shorts, debate whether to compete at all, then get myself (sweating on a cool day) to the start area. I watched my closest competitor Carl Moore take off 2 minutes ahead. Convincing myself that I might just be able to walk around to a few controls before bagging it, I drank more water and took off, vowing to be extremely conservative. I'd planned to stick on or close to trails, keep in constant touch with the map (thumb compass pointing to my exact location always), and be ready to collapse on a big trail or walk back to the finish at any moment if need be. Selecting the most bombproof attack points, and sure and simple routes regardless of the time factor involved, seemed the sensible thing to do.

Carl was last seen climbing a hill far ahead of me at control 2, and thereafter the only competitor seen was Pat Albright on a different course. I did all those things we're taught or pick up with lots of experience, such as frequent checking of the compass, matching features passed with the map, verifying directions after trail turns or junctions, using handrails, etc. Otherwise, using not just one navigational tool on each leg, but many. At the mid-point control I stopped for water and told the Air Force Search & Rescue person my name, and suggested that he might be done for the day, since I was last out.

The next leg was the cleverly designed killer leg—almost 1200 meters with no ready handrail, except a hard-to-follow contour. The course designer Scott Donald told me later that he had set the Green course up to make this the premier leg. It was later found that an earlier, easier leg undid many. One look at this leg caused me to reject the direct route, trying to hit a tiny grove of trees on a faint foot trail after the long, featureless open forest trek. The alternative, a long, looping jeep trail that involved an added 700 meters, but with the safety of a ready handrail, two side roads, and good compass checkpoints at the bends looked promising. I worried about possibly passing or undershooting the side trail connection with the jeep road, so I carefully pace-counted and timed myself. For the first time. I even jogged this leg, and was pleased to nail the road-trail junction and then the control!

Somewhat elated, my male ego then overrode common sense when I encountered Pat Albright and attempted to run up a steep hillside in front of her! My body instantly told my brain NO WAY, and I found myself following her around instead of up over the 6 contours of the 12-contour river bluff I didn't need to climb. My legs and digestive system thanked my brain (and Pat) for compromising!

So finally to the Finish—but no one was there but the finish timer! People were off having lunch, comparing routes, and having fun, so I dragged on back to the parking lot and changed my shorts again, thankful to have just finished. John Sincock, sitting in the next car, yelled over that I'd had a good day, I quipped back something disrespectful, and questioned how long he'd been sitting there. He responded that Carl Moore, Knut Olson, and Doug Sprugel weren't in yet—and he'd taken my picture crossing the finish line. Somewhat confused, I stumbled back to the finish to watch my chase start competitors arrive, and it suddenly struck me that, wonder of wonders (or as my many friends say—an outright fluke) I'd become the WASHINGTON STATE CHAMP! (Don't ask how many were in my class—we're focusing on lessons learned here.)

Since that time, I've adopted the I'M SICK TECHNIQUE or style, with very good results, at least compared to the old aggressive style: competing at my own fitness level, not some other competitor's; trying to outthink the course designer by using obscure handrails and simplifying the map; treating even the easiest leg like it might be the killer; using the terrain, and not letting it use me; thumbing the map like I'm supposed to; and knowing how to get back quickly if DNF seems the optimum solution.

Now, to September 1992 and the Washington State Champs at Cle Elum Ridge. The same new technique was used here, but this time I'd not done any training or even running for a year, attended very few meets, and was on penicillin for severely clogged sinuses. The open forest and very dry conditions allowed almost bee-line shots between controls, even through mapped dark green fight areas. The weather was perfect.

The first day I walked the course, and my only problem was a loss of focus when the male ego kicked in again. Karen Lachance appeared ahead of me walking on the leg between controls 4 and 5. I tried to RUN by her and get out of sight before she could trail me into the control. Of course, I could barely breathe after that exertion, and had to walk slowly on the next leg, with the thinking process in neutral. So I overshot the next control by two minutes, and found Karen walking past me as I returned down HER backtrail to get the control. Such a humbling sport!

The second day I also walked, and had only a minor problem in focusing when I missed finding the end of a vague ridge top, an exceedingly poor attack point. By awards ceremony time, I hadn't even checked the entry list or results for either day—so, when Carl Coger of B.C. won the blue ribbon in my class, I was perfectly set up for the surprise result—you've guessed it—I'm once again the WASHINGTON STATE CHAMP!

Does the I'm Sick Technique work, or what? Might it work for you? I now always carry with me my COMPASS—that is: Compromise on speed vs. accuracy, Outwit the course designer, Map read constantly, Pace myself, Assess options on routes, Spare body so brain can work, Seek easiest way to finish!

Good luck in the forest!

ROGAINE PLANNING – Plus an Invitation

Sunset: 8:04 pm Pacific Daylight Time (PDT). Sunrise: 6:25 am PDT. But what are the EENT and BMNT times? Must call the Army or US Weather Bureau. And Moonrise is 2:57 AM, Moonset 5:42 AM according to the Farmer's Almanac. Hmm! Is this data accurate for Latitude 47 degrees, 15 minutes N., Longitude 120 degrees, 30' W on August 14th night and 15th morning, 1993?

Well, you wonder—who cares? The answer is: The rogaine course planners now, and soon the 100-plus participants in the second 24-hour rogaine to be held at Table Mountain in Washington State. Again, you might ask—"So what? It's always cloudy and rainy there, so who'll ever see the moon, much less the sun, during a 24-hour event in the mountains?" The answer is, hopefully: This is Eastern Washington, in the summer, at elevations over 5000 feet, and in fairly open forest. Visibility should be excellent, with only scattered clouds. Temperatures expected from 50 to 90 degrees F., some deer and elk, no grazing cattle, and lots of other wildlife to enjoy.

Your friendly US Forest Service has approved the use of this Wenatchee National Forest area at Table Mountain, after many phone calls and a detailed permit application. We have thrashed out the impact problems of over one hundred campers and a lot of cars going into this area—to a one-time use no-facility camping area. Bring your own water bottles and purifying stuff. Porta-toilets will be provided, plus a continuous meal after 6 PM Saturday through the event end at noon Sunday.

How to Do It

For those considering organizing a ROGAINE soon, the following planning details are offered here for guidance. Much of this is based on Keg Good's Lessons Learned About Rogaines notes of July 8th, 1992, from her experiences, plus lessons from events in Canada and the rogaines in Washington.

Get a sponsoring club! You'll need their resources—including about 40 or so Orienteering marker controls, experienced volunteers who can unerringly locate your kitchentable-selected control features using outdated 1:24000 to 1:69,000 scale topo maps to flag them; insurance coverage from USOF or another sports body; and the logistics personnel who will willingly and faithfully organize and set up the administrative and food facilities needed at the base camp—which I like to call the Hash House (HH), the way Australians do.

Get permissions. Contact the landowners, Forest Service, local sheriff, Search and Rescue teams, and any groups which may have reservations for events in the area.

Get every map available for the area of interest. For a 24-hour event, the area should be about 10 by 10 km, or 100 square km.; varied and forested topography preferred. The USGS 7 1/2 minute quads are most useful in our area, and the Forest Service fire road maps usually show most the drivable roads. It is very important that the parking and HH be reachable by a good-surface road so that all participants can drive in. Alternative parking areas and bus or shuttle service, or even using 4WD vehicles might work, but add many problems that could lead to a less-than-successful event.

Make a preliminary plan for control placement, using a good distribution of controls throughout the area. Since this is a score-course event, the control locations are usually given score values based on some cleverly designed scheme of point assignment.

Planning the Course

For a 24-hour event, plan to use about 34 to 40 controls (scale back accordingly for 6, 8, or 12-hour) with a score distribution of: 5 at 20 pts, 5 at 30, 8 at 40, 7 at 50, 6 at 60, 5 at 80, and 4 at 100. Challenging, but fun, sets the proper tone; you want to give both the ultra-marathoners and the family day-hikers planning and execution challenges within their diverse capabilities. The score values are assigned based on distance from the HH, distance from adjacent controls, climb involved from adjacent points, difficulty of navigation in the immediate area, scenic value of feature (yes, you can do some tour-guiding to you most scenic spots by assigning high values).

Be careful in assigning point values around the HH in all directions, so that no part of the map is obviously the best area to pick up the highest score quickly. The course planners will find enormous satisfaction watching the mass start teams scattering to all points of the compass!

Controls should be no closer than one kilometer to each other, if possible. Also, good planners don't locate controls right on roads, main trails, or often-visited features where other visitors in the area might remove your control bags before (or worse—during) the event. The Australian Course Planners Manual suggests using an offset control description to safeguard your markers where necessary—something like: Top of hill (viewpoint), then 30 meters W 270 degrees in dense brush. This offset should be used sparingly, since at this scale map, the feature might be hard enough to identify without question if it has no marker visible. Also, remember that night navigation is even trickier, and without a visible reflectorized marker to seek out, that hidden marker might take hours to locate!

Once a suitable HH is located, I try to put relatively low-value (20 or 30 pts) controls on easy features near good trails or roads in at least 5 different directions from the start. Just beyond each of these, I try to have two high-pointers (50 to 80 pts) to attract teams that way. Since the best route-planners are looking at contouring and the climb involved very closely, so the planner should, too. Next, I select the most challenging and distance features. I put those four 100 pointers initially at the four far corners of the 10x10 km "playing field", and offer the challenge to the elite teams to get them all in the 24 hours. If the essential water is set out in bottles on or near drivable roads, these become controls themselves, with appropriate score points. Otherwise, participants may unwisely choose to ignore them.

Make It Fun for All

The ideal course, in my view, will give the family day-hikers one or two easy loop routes that will gain them maybe 400 points in two easy day-hikes, say 12 to 6 PM and then 7-12 Noon. However, the most elite teams, like Peter Gagarin and Fred Pilon (World Rogaine Veteran champs, 4th overall), moving at 5 to 6 km per hour for maybe 20 hours of walking/running, will most likely reach most of the controls. (I'd be very embarrassed if some team got them all and came in several hours early!)

As in Orienteering events, you must field-check each control location early, and determine that the location can be found using the provided map, from any compass direction, with due consideration to night navigation problems and safety. Its point value must be calculated vs. all the other controls. Sample routes can then be done by map-study, to see if it is too easy to find optimal routes for high scores. When control bags are ready to be set, the people doing the placements should be using the actual map for the event, and the control descriptions in final draft form. A different person from the original field checker should be sent, to avoid some of the navigational errors possible. The marker must be hung where it can be seen at night, and tied (I hope) so that animals or 40-knot winds won't remove it before the event. Deer seem to love to chew on tie-strings, even nylon, if there is enough body sweat to give a salty taste to them.

At each control location, an Intention Sheet is also tied in place, along with the control punch to mark the control card carried by the rogaine team. When the team punches in, they must also sign in, show the current time, and indicate where they INTEND to go next. These intention sheets are a safety feature in case of lost teams, an attempt to police the rule that teams must not separate on the course, a means of friendly communication to other competitive teams that you beat them there, and perhaps a help to confused teams as to where it might be best to go next! After the event, when these intention sheets are recovered, a detailed spreadsheet could be made up to show each team's arrival time at all visited controls. (An enormous job, but some people like lots of data!)

They'll Get Hungry

Food planning and service are historically a very important part of a rogaine. Although teams are responsible for their own on-trail nourishment and water, the Hash House environment is one of recovery, tall-story telling, camaraderie, refreshment, ravishing hunger, and a need for hot food in large quantities whenever a team arrives back. The planners can figure about $5.00 or more per person for the food budget, and should expect to prepare hot soup, perhaps stew, drinks, and provide for self-service preparation a wide variety of fruits, vegetables, breads, crackers, and other filling items. Luxury products like baked goods and beer/wine might be offered for individual purchase, if you have volunteers willing to take care of it. A large food tent separated from the administration tent or area is needed. We always plan for rain at some time during the event, so shelter is important. Don't forget the sanitation facilities, extra water, first aid gear, and the backhaul of garbage.

With pre-registration, you should have very few day-of-event changes. A self-scoring punch card is used, so the organizers must only verify the punch count and double-check the addition as the teams finish to determine final scores and awards. Usually, rogaine awards, token in nature, are often hand-crafted and representative of the local area. In addition, if sponsors have donated prizes, these can be grouped and winners allowed to choose one from the "pile" and all left-over prizes are given based on a drawing from the control-cards of finishing teams that are still present at the awards ceremony.

By the way, a rogaine is usually attended by several teams who must leave soon after the finish—so awards should be handled quickly. To expedite this, and for safety purposes, a very high penalty is imposed for late finishers. At least 10 points per minute is recommended, with a no award or perhaps a zero score penalty after 30 to 60 minutes late.

I Thought You'd Never Ask

If your team would like to challenge the Table Mountain Rogaine, you may send in an application form now, using the USOF or ONA generic form, or even a letter. Send your entry to the Sammamish Orienteering Club, PO Box 3682, Bellevue, WA 98009. Entry fees to be announced will cover maps, food, prizes, USFS application and user fees, printing and postage, and site facility rentals. You may pre-register now for the Men's, Women's, Mixed, Masters (over 40), or Group sections. Include ages of all teammates. Select the 12-hour option if you prefer. Further information will be mailed to your team's address about one month before the event. Although the Table Mountain area north of Ellensburg, WA, is now embargoed to you, we can't stop you from ordering the Green Trails map at $2.50 each of Liberty, No.210 and Thorp, No.242 from Pioneer Maps, 1645 140th Ave NE, Bellevue, WA 98005—or sneakily perusing the USGS quads in advance. My experience is that this does little to help even the most dedicated competitive team, but at least you'll be able to estimate your driving time, and figure how to get to the event area in advance.

Please call or write the author or this publication for more help in YOUR rogaine planning!

REDDICK'S ROGAINE RUMINATIONS

Twenty-four hour Rogaine events often produce memories that stick with you long after the blisters are healed and the fatigue is forgotten. And, fortunately or not, you as a competitor have at least one partner with whom to share the glory or divide the blame.

Rogaine organizers also share such memories!

Preparing for the first Rogaine in the US back in 1989, Doug Caley and others from the King County Search and Rescue (SAR) group joined Washington State's Nisqually O-Club volunteers in doing preliminary field work, marking and vetting control locations in the two months prior to the May event in the Cascade Mountains. The event was held in open evergreen forest and rough mountain pasture-land in the Wenatchee National Forest south of Cle Elum, and to the northeast of Mt. Rainier. This Manastash area has elevations ranging from 3800 to 5800 feet, and still had pockets of snow in north-facing re-entrants and shaded spots in March and April.

Doug and I (yes, two intrepid and highly experienced navigators) set out on a loop trip to check several pre-selected control sites for suitability, and to hang ribbons to indicate the placement of regular Orienteering control flags later, plus Intention Sheets. (An intention sheet is a pre-printed sign-in log placed at each control for safety and verification purposes. Each member of the Rogaine team signs in there, reports the time of arrival, and shows the number of the next control they "intend" to visit. Use of this sheet discourages violation of the rule that team members must stick together—NOT: "Al, you climb that 12-contour hill for #101, while I wait here and redo my foot bandages!")

Rogaine maps commonly are 1:24,000 to 1:60,000 scale standard topographic maps, with almost no updating. The control locations must be selected to be clearly identifiable on the ground and, while they do not necessarily have to be features shown on the map, the surrounding area must be fairly accurately mapped, and no "bingo controls." This is particularly important in these events, since the course setter and control hanger must remember that the control may be approached from any direction, and in the classic 24-hour event, this may be at 2 AM, no moon, and during a rainstorm! All control bags used were marked on each face with reflective tape, hung high and clear of vegetation to permit 360° viewing where possible. A few survived wind-whipping and nibbling by deer—could moth balls in the hems of the markers help?

We were using the "Control Vetter Card" for the first time (shown at right). These cards were prepared and given out to the field checkers, with instructions to verify the location, map accuracy, suitability, and scenic value of the location, while flagging it. Also, checkers were asked to evaluate the potential point value of the control, ranging from 20 to 100 points, per the 3 scaled items shown. In this example, the values

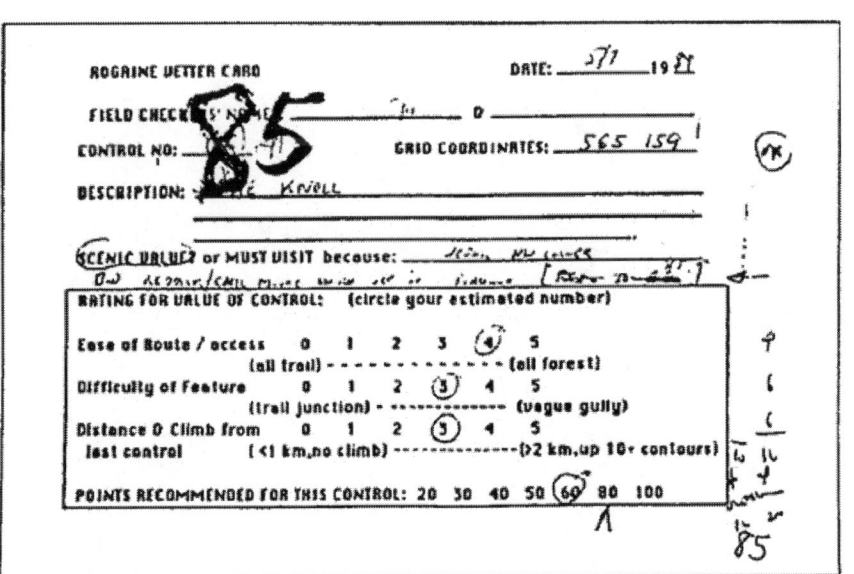

Published in *Orienteering North America* June 1993 issue.

called for a score of 60 or maybe 80, compared to all other controls ratings. This control was finally given a value of 80 and control number 85, weighting the scenic value slightly more than the distance and difficulty. The Rogaine organizer can certainly be biased toward being a tour guide to the best parts of the "playing field!"

Doug carried a large backpack, and had a radio to test communications with another SAR team and the base station in his truck, and to check the proposed relay site. After a lunch stop near #58, we approached the first of three key hilltops about 1 km northeast of the Hash House (Aussie term for the base camp). The northern and southern hilltops were to be regular control locations, while the center one was to be the secret, location of the "lost Rogaine team," which was an add-on optional adventure game to this Rogaine. The idea was to give the competing rogainers, plus the 6 SAR teams supporting us, a puzzle in figuring where the lost team might be, given their log times and intended destinations at the 18 controls (of 45) which they had visited (simulated) before they became lost. One stationary SAR Team would be camped at this center hilltop, manning a radio relay, and be the "lost Rogaine team." Bonus points were to be given for those who found them (6 teams of 55 actually did!). So the bracketing controls at 82 and 84 were critical.

At this first hilltop area (see map, #82), we climbed up a steep ridge in low overcast and near white-out conditions, found the supposedly highest point, then found a suitable tree to tie long engineer tape ribbons. Suddenly we were hit with a swirling snow squall, which brought out the hats and parkas. In about 10 minutes it subsided, and we started on to the central hilltop (see 5177 trig point). After about 50 meters, we found the terrain rising sharply again, much too soon! A few more minutes found us on top of a much higher hill, obviously the one we thought we were on minutes before!

Navigationally embarrassed, Doug and I marked this new #82. and then retreated back to remove the flagging at the erroneous one. Congratulating ourselves on saving what would have been a major error in the event, we moved on to the central hilltop, where the weather cleared enough for us to see downward in all directions for this relay site and "lost Rogaine team" spot. After flagging this, we trudged northward to control location #84. where we sought out the highest point on a rocky spur for our flagging. We used both pace-counting and timing to check the distance, but accuracy over almost one kilometer of forested, rocky terrain is not great. The surrounding terrain didn't look just right, so to be SURE we had the right spot, we decided to follow a re-entrant southwestward down the steep, forested hillside to a creek junction, where I had hung flagging for #43 the previous fall. Working our way down this hillside proved very difficult, since snow remained in drifts up to 3 feet deep in spots, with the only clear route being right in the running stream bed in the re-entrant. Sure enough, when we reached the bottom, there was the flagging at the stream junction—thus confirming our precise navigation—NOT!

One week prior to the event, our organizers' team was out making final control/intention sheet placements. Carl Moore reported back that #84 flagging was not in the right place, but he'd hung the control there anyway, and placed the flagging at the mapped location. With some disbelief, I went back, reflecting that resetting a Rogaine marker often takes 2 hours plus 1000 feet of climb, contrasted with Orienteering course correction of minutes and a few contours. Carl was right, of course, and with much chagrin I moved the marker, then sat down to study the map to see why the exhausting snowdrift descent hadn't verified the right spot.

As you may figure out yourself, looking at the map, it was a parallel error of the most insidious kind. Can you find it? Our flagging was some 200 meters off! (Clue: look at the shape of the re-entrant.)

Talking about control placements—two others in this event were somewhat controversial—both involving fear of wet feet. The first one, at the end of Lost Lake, was to be set at the junction of two streams and the lake edge. This area was under 2-3 feet of snow when the marker was hung, but by event time it was slushy, marshy ground, with a stream delta there. Several teams reported having to wade to punch in, but Debbie Newell found a feet-dry approach on Sunday—via logs.

The second one, control #34, a re-entrant junction lying in a meadow-like open area, was a use of an implied feature that Graham Foley of Australia has recommended be used for more challenging map-reading. Can you see this junction? This area was also very boggy when Wanda Howlett approached to hang the marker. Being thoughtful and considerate, she hung the reflectorized control in plain sight at the first dry point to the northeast. However, a few teams who approached from certain directions, and those arriving at night, could not see it readily, and had to do an area search to find the marker. Extremely wet feet—as well as bad tempers, resulted. Please note that an area search in Rogaining, including just the terrain inside the 6 mm control circle on the map, equals about 4 acres or 1.6 hectares on a 1:24,000 map. Imagine trying to search THAT in partial moonlight!

So for all you potential Rogaine organizers—good luck in trying to arrange your 100-square-kilometer "playing fields" with deliberate, not accidental, navigational challenges. You just can't be too careful, or skimp on independent vetting for either Orienteering or Rogaining!

TABLE MOUNTAIN ROGAINE

The 1993 Table Mountain Rogaine, the First Western Hemisphere Championships of Rogaining (officially unsanctioned by the International Rogaining Federation), August 14-15, 1993, was attended by 75 hardy competitors, with 32 official teams and 2 unofficial ones. The final standings are at the end of this report. The random and noteworthy observations by some of the organizers and participants follow. Most teams did not choose team names, so we've dropped them from this report—but we must mention the jewel of a name—the HUFFIN PUFFINS, Dan Ellsworth and Jackie Bergt from Anchorage, AK! The top teams in points achieved remarkable distances, climbs, and speeds, with the overall winner going 80.7 km in 22:55 hours with almost 10,700 feet of climb. Every team certainly had a physical and mental challenge in executing their own chosen route plan at their own fitness level in this tough terrain. Many, many different route choices were made by the teams to all parts of the map, with every one of the 46 controls visited at least three times, with the average being 12 teams visiting. More teams stayed out after sunset and even after Ending Evening Civil Twilight (see chart) than at any other known Western Hemisphere rogaine to date! It won't be long before most teams will seek out the 24-hour challenge, and will even start practicing night navigation before major rogaines.

Our low temperature was 41.6°F at 4 AM, with highs ranging up to almost 60 degrees during the overcast, hint-of-rain daylight hours—just about perfect conditions for this event. Clearer skies would have produced views in the distance of Mt. Rainier, Mt. Adams, Mt. Stewart, and the eastern Washington plateau, which might have distracted these teams from their appointed rounds. Surrounding valley views were reportedly OK, though. Vegetation and trails were dry and mud-free, but deadfall in parts of the forest made off-trail travel slow. The ten gallons of water placed at each of 6 water controls for 75 participants was overkill for a cool weather event—only about 3 gallons was used at the most-visited ones. Had it been the expected 80°F or more and sunny, this water would have been about right. Most teams carried two or three bottles per person, and refilled at the water controls (which had score values). The paper cups provided there were hardly used.

Could our US Forest Service expect any more than to have almost 80 people, US and foreign citizens alike, tramping off-trail through rugged terrain searching for wolf shit (or scat, dung, feces, sign, or doo-doo, if you prefer)? And we found some! This has been duly reported with grid coordinates to the Leavenworth Ranger District Gray Wolf Study project leader. So this long-gone creature may be coming back into this State. We hope to hear more, later.

Should both teams have been disqualified when one team member loaned a flashlight to another team to allow a person to return to the Hash House without stumbling in the dark? A direct violation of Rule 3. The soft-hearted director allowed this, and yes, Mark, you're getting your flashlight back. And can a women's team still be one if a late-arriving male person joins it on the second morning? How can all dinner food for 80 people be gone by midnight, when the well-warned caterers brought enough for 100 people? Is it really true that someone was seen having 6 bowls of soup? Did someone clean out the remaining soup at 2 AM by filling a thermos for their packs? How come the pasta and most of the requested veggies got left out of the menu—they're cheap and easy to fix! Can totally knackered trenchermen rogainers restrain themselves when finally dragging back within smelling distance of hot food? The dear answer to the last question is NO! But the issued PowerBars got many teams through the whole event, and most swore by them, not at them. We quote one team: "We couldn't have finished without them!" (Yes, Powerfood Inc., we're doing more of these rogaines all over, and we know your toll-free number.) Hot dogs (specifically not requested for this rogaine menu) proved to be the lifesaver for several teams, including, perhaps, the overall winner. Dave Tallent, the volunteer night chef and Head of the Complaint Department, performed yeomanlike service in handling this tough part of the rogaine (but no one promised it would be easy—as all were warned by a cartoon in the rules).

Published in *Orienteering North America* September 1993 issue.

One large buck elk with velvet 15-inch antlers was sighted on Sunday near Control 61 during pickup. Many other elk, deer, grouse, squirrels, chipmunks, hawks, etc. were also reported. A few cattle were loose all over the Southeast part of the map—in violation of their grazing permit! This added to the color of the area. That gray wolf shit was spotted on Diamond Head by Susan McGovern, Wenatchee, and Megan Schneebaum of Washington, D.C. The perturbed pregnant porcupine resident at Rider's Cabin was not reported seen by any rogainers. An eagle's nest was spotted in a snag enroute to control #81. An old crashed airplane was found along Drop Creek. Two teams camped out, and another (the Women's 24-hour winners) chose a 3-hour "death march" back to the HH after dark, were heard laughing about it in their tent at 1 AM, and were rewarded by fresh coffee and great pancakes for breakfast!

If you camped right next to the Hash House food tent with its accompanying generator and lights, you were only a few steps from the campfire and breakfast, but had lots of generator noise, lights, and loud conversations going to keep you awake all night! The only reported injury, except to navigational-skill pride, was a rogainer who reported a bee-sting from an angry swarm when he walked over an underground nest between the Hash House food and administrative areas-—a deadfall area traversed numerous times by the organizers over 3 days without incident.

The mass start was video-taped, and shows about 1/4 of the teams going south, most going north to #81 (9) and #22 (8), and 6 teams east to #21. This is exactly what the course designer, Dave Enger, had hoped to achieve in setting a tough-to-figure course. One team successfully lost their punch card and one map. Rather than start them off again with a zero score, we accepted their sworn affidavit that they had actually visited some controls during that 7:42 hour hike—pending confirmation after the event by close scrutiny of the intention sheet entries. Another team (medalists) left behind their pencils (too much weight?) while dog-legging into one control, and claim to have scratched their entry on the intention sheet with a rock! Close examination of the sheet reveals what may be a "10" scratched in the Team block underneath another team's later entry! Disqualification is still possible for up to a year, while we carefully study the matter. We did find one control bag badly mangled at #31, and the intention sheet torn down, trampled, and partially eaten at #57 one week later.

One team logged in using elapsed time, and maybe Eastern Daylight Time and/or Central Daylight Time driving the results compilation committee absolutely nuts in trying to make sense of what really happened. Or maybe they carried sundials—and we did have overcast skies! Next time, we will specify local time for all entries, and insist that all watches be adjusted to the announced time hack! Another team often logged in using the team number of one of their spouses—again, another puzzle to solve. Most teams showed their actual routes on black and white maps provided, which were displayed at the Hash House, and later mailed to all participants. Silly answers given to questions asked: Nick: What is the difference between the 24-hour event and the 12in24 hour event? Answer: Twelve hours. Sandy: What is the little waterproof J. L. Darling Corporation notebook for? Answer: To write in. Write what? Answer: Anything you like. (The "Rite-in-the-Rain" map and intention sheet paper, and intention boards came from them.)

Only a few pithy comments were noted on the Intention Sheets: "We like the blue sky to the east"; "What a view—worth the drive"; "Kick off the rowdies [Lion Rock]"; "Lost map already"; "Team 37 put wrong hour!"; "What's a rogaine? No one knows. What's a henway? Oh, a couple of pounds!"; "At least 80 points [at #81]!"; "Next time I will go for a 24 minutes option at most!!!"; "[We're] first to #83"; "Ridiculous! No need be this difficult [At #104, which 5 worthy teams chose to include in their route! Even our vetter didn't like this one, due to the punishing climb in and out of Wilson Creek valley.]"; "The scree was pretty rough!"; "This is cool metelo". We invite all participants to send in further comments to the Sammamish Orienteering Club on how to improve the next rogaine.

The Meet Director admitted to a feeling of dismay and impending defeat Saturday night when early reports came in that the "Gagarin" team was signing in at controls all over the northern loop, while other teams mentioned that the southern loop was being wrapped up by the Gagarin team! They were doing it all in one 12-hour period, and were going to come in about midnight Saturday to eat, sleep, and go home wondering why they'd bothered to come! It wasn't until exactly 12:52 AM Sunday when a team came in to eat that the truth dawned that those were two different teams! What a relief! We somehow forgot to give out the Waltzing Matilda (you'll come rogaining, Matilda with me) music to those around the campfire Saturday night.

The Table Mountain Rogaine map preparation story, requested by several future organizers: Preparing the course for an elite team entry caused the need for three USGS maps to get a 90+ km course length. Since each map cost $2.50 and they are hard to obtain in quantity, we needed to produce our own map. Laser color printing at prices under $2.00 in quantity dictated the 11" x 17" map size, which led to the 1:36,000 scale, or a reduction of the USGS maps to 66% of original size. Test printing at Kinko's proved marginal, since color quality among the three maps was inconsistent, and the vegetation boundaries on the Reecer Creek (Southern map) were poorly defined. So we went to Pacific Color Labs at Green Lake in Seattle, and they suggested that best quality would result from the following steps: Photograph master onto 35mm film; digitally scan the film; put onto CD ROM and then computer manipulate (enhance) digitally the portions of the map needing help, and then reduce to final size. Then, go digitally into the laser printer (no new optical process), and print out the 100 color copies. Prices quoted for the map: 35mm slide $6.00, computer manipulate $15.00, 100 each 11x17 color laser prints @ $1.50. Actual price per copy charged was $0.99 (what a deal, and 3-day service, too)! for a total cost of $129.84. With all the test runs and working copies, plus waterproof paper at $0.15 each, led to a per-map cost of about $1.70, with 20 or so left-over maps to use for promotion of Rogaining throughout the US—er, the Western Hemisphere! End of map report, except to note for you purists that the final map scale came out at 1:37,600, due to the margins needed on the 11x17—which we didn't anticipate.

GENERAL ROGAINING NEWS: The International Rogaining Federation is looking for a venue for the next World Championships—any ideas? Like to volunteer to organize it? Call or write soon. We are also seeking ideas on how an organizer should prepare or plan for an elite team attending his/her event. By adding 20% to the maximum course length? By providing a handicap in time, or extra controls for just the elite? By not worrying about it? By imposing the 100-pound pack rule? Any thoughts? A group of rogainers may be referred to hereafter as a QUEST of rogainers, which is perhaps more appropriate than a VENERY of rogainers—the association with a romantic adventure is better than that of a new form of VD!

We'd like to thank our sponsors—K-Swiss shoes, PowerBar, and REI stores nationwide, but particularly the Bellevue, Federal Way, Lynnwood, and Seattle REI stores, who contributed a large part of their monthly promotion budgets each to support us. Also thanks should go to all the following: the course setters—Kevin and Virginia Finney, John Sincock, Mark Howlett, and Ken Lew. Believe it or not, some of the controls were flown in from Seattle by Mike Schuh to our vetter when the schedule got tight! And that indefatigable vetter, Kent Verbeck. The aforementioned course designer and also vetter, Dave Enger, the Awards Person Jana Urbanova (of Czech O' fame), the night chef Dave Tallent, water bearers Peter Bonek and Eric Bone, Rick Hood for ideas and the results board work, the COC and EOC clubs for equipment and local knowledge help (particularly Will Sperry). The caterer—Bill Burvee and partner, who did a marvelous job, particularly since they're used to serving three short meals of barbecued cow meat in large quantities to outdoor eaters at $25.00 a head, not one 20-hour meal to rogainers at $10.00! Cascade Trophy of Lynnwood did the beautiful medals and the many award ribbons. Thanks also to all of you who were part of 'The one-control pickup,' plus Peter Golde who helped on the after-event course cleanup and this article. Ken Lew assisted in the results report preparation. The Sammamish Orienteering Club was your host.

Thanks go the Luci Bull and the Cle Elum Ranger Station folks, US Forest Service, for fast, courteous service and the flora and fauna information, although we didn't like the required but very expensive permit. Also thanks to the Australian folks who invented this sport, and provided much guidance and ideas over the past 5 years, and to the International Rogaining Federation for politely remaining mute to informally sanction this First Western Hemisphere Championships of Rogaining!

ROGAINING PET THEORIES

Some of my pet theories, worthy of serious criticism or argument:

The best team at the event should reach all but one control in the time limit, given ideal weather and a quality map. Without this, teams either haven't enough challenge, or at the other extreme, every team is pursuing a different course, with almost no comparison possible in looking at results.

Economy of effort for the organisers. Minimize area used and number of controls placed, while also maximising the enjoyment of the participants. This also should allow more careful checking and vetting of controls to insure an error-free course.

Encourage, lobby for, and support the 24-hour event as the CLASSIC rogaine, with anything less a means of drawing more people into the sport and getting them confident enough to do the endurance and night-navigation involved. Too many 3-hour events in the USA are being called 'Rogaines'—which I don't mind now, but hope to see some minimum standard for this name in the future. I propose 8 hours as a minimum, unless specifically advertised as a training event.

Insist that all organisers include water controls (not just unscored drop points), as an essential part of any course. These can be natural water sources, public or private fixed facilities, or water jugs at the control. Since route choice, navigation, and a carefully vetted site are all involved with every site on a rogaine map, I feel very strongly that water resupply must be carefully planned and some minimum level provided for any event.

Food service and the Hash House environment. Probably second only to fair controls unerringly placed as mapped as the most remembered part of any rogaine—and probably most critical to the event's overall success. Food always seems to be the most expensive thing in any budget, too. It would be of great value to any organizer to have a food list, equipment list, stall requirements, sample budget, and recommended ways of meeting the needs of, say, 50,100, 200, and 300 people. Specific food items will vary by country, but most rogainers seek basically the same things (with variety) to consume when returning to the Hash House.

Publicity and advertising media for specific events and rogaining in general. *Orienteering North America* [USA orienteering magazine] have done great by including a special section in the monthly Schedule of Events for rogaines, and doing frequent 'In The Long Run' feature articles in the magazine. My advertising for the Table Mountain rogaine, including display ads in several regional and national magazines, flyers in sports and hiking stores, e-mail and orienteering event flyers, etc., gave positive results only when preceded or followed by face-to-face or telephone contact. It seems that interested participants have to be personally invited and encouraged (challenged, threatened, cajoled, or dragged along in the car) to get them to their first rogaine. This often results in them never being seen again, but much more often wanting to attend every rogaine possible. Some even liked them so much they volunteer to help!

Here's a debatable one: I think no "nest" of three controls anywhere on the map (possible exception—right next to the Hash House) should have a total score value of less than 100, nor more than 200 points. This is to make route planning that much harder in trying to achieve an optimum score for time travelled.

Bob's formula for calculating checkpoint scores is:

[km to HH]*2.0 + [km to closest checkpoint]*2.0 + [km to 2nd closest checkpoint]*2.0 + [elevation gain to nearest checkpoint (in feet)]*0.05 + [elevation gain to 2nd nearest]*0.05 + [difficulty (1-5)]*3.0 + [km to nearest trail]*20.0 + [tour factor - scenic or plug variable (0-2)]* 10.0.

Part of a privately circulated letter dated September 30, 1993.

INTERVIEW

BOB REDDICK, Washington State, USA

Bob is the current US Orienteering Federation Rogaine Committee Chairman and directed the first rogaine in the USA.

Age: 59

Occupation: Real Estate Sales. Retired US Army Ordnance Officer. Electrical Engineering and Operations Research degrees.

How Started Rogaining

After moving from 'couch potato' and doubles tennis player to orienteering in 1987, found article in *Orienteering North America* on rogaining and heard of Murray Foubister's rogaine at Kamloops, B.C. coming in May '88. Persuaded Knut Olson (older, US national O' champ, and with endless endurance) to partner with me. After 4 months of intensive walking/running/orienteering training, I was barely able to keep up with him—but we survived a memorable 24-hour event and I was hooked! My wife Pat also enjoys rogaining and orienteering events and people, but not doing the courses.

Rogaining Achievements

Very low-key effort compared to Andy Newson and Kitty Jones in Calgary, Foubister in Kamloops, and Neil Phillips internationally in publicizing, sponsoring, and directing events. But with much help from those stalwarts and local orienteering club members, I organized and directed the first US rogaine in Washington State in May 1989. Competed in several 24-hour rogaines in Canada, and Rick Hood's 6-hour events at Drunken Charlie Lake near Seattle each year. Usually intentionally stayed out all night, and never was warm enough to sleep for more than 2 hours, in spite of fatigue. Partnered with Neil Phillips at the B.C. rogaine near Kamloops in 1989. (His slow jog was my all-out sprint!) Tried to get to First World Champs in Australia with my wife, Pat, but low-budget military aerial hitchhiking plan failed. Helped Bruce McAlister run the Dancing Lady Rogaine at White Pass area, Washington in August 1991. Recently directed First Western Hemisphere Championships of Rogaining at Table Mountain, WA, August 1993. Have written many rogaining articles and reports for *ONA* and *Bearing 315* publications and *IRF* newsletters.

Biggest navigational accomplishments so far, besides getting feet and lungs able to last more than an hour, were winning state orienteering championship and relay champ in 1989, and again in 1992.

Now in early planning stage for the Sasquatch Rogaine at Mt. St. Helens (yes, the active volcano!). All sasquatches, bigfeet, yetis, and almas will have free entry to compete.

What I Like About Rogaining

The whole concept! Particularly the partnership or team aspect, which helps keep up your motivation to excel on the course, provides a witness to your navigational and physical successes (and someone to blame besides yourself for those inevitable errors), and differentiates it from orienteering—which I also enjoy. Surprised to find how much I enjoyed and was good at night navigation, the prospect of which seems to deter many from entering the 24-hour classic rogaine section. The feeling that you are really competing against the clock and your own skill and endurance limits, with the planning part almost as

Published in *IRF Bulletin #2*, 1994.

important as the execution. No DNFs or disqualifications for teams, so everyone has a result that is most meaningful in comparison to what they tried to achieve—not to what other teams did! And not to forget the Hash House camaraderie, which adds so much to the events.

Special Gear

In preparing for that first rogaine, I researched everything. Took Exceed sports drink mix in packets to make up along the way with water from creeks and beaver ponds. We used less than half of it—but it helped since we made no Hash House stop and had just a few granola bars for solid food. Layered clothing, no cotton items, and using the "10-pound pack rule" (I invented this one), we found ourselves well-equipped for most eventualities. Least-carried but most-needed item is a ground pad for sitting and sleeping! I now have a very light, self-inflatable one. Often carried or picked up along the trail a hiking stick adjustable for the terrain, which was extremely useful for steep uphills and downhills, and critical for swift creek crossings. I understand hiking with two adjustable poles (like in cross-country skiing) is coming on big in Europe now.

Rogaining Story

My most memorable experience not already reported in prior issues of *ONA* was a bit of night navigation at the 1989 BC Research Forest Reserve rogaine with Steve Cockle near Maple Ridge, British Columbia. Steve and I had decided to stay out the full 24-hours, mainly because we weren't doing too well navigationally or physically, and were far from the base camp at dark. So we attacked a control on a narrow spur, but missed it (being on a parallel spur). We broke for a rest about midnight—tried to sleep on a trail—after 2 hours or so, we got too cold, so got up and re-tried for the missed control. Coming down the ridgeline from the top in the dark through heavy underbrush, I found in my headlamp's beam a large downed tree (Douglas fir?) pointing our way, which would allow us to walk above the wet and nasty underbrush for about 100 feet. With Steve behind, I stepped carefully along this 3-foot diameter hulk, weaving among the infrequent branch limbs, until my light showed what looked like the top of our tree caught between two stumps in the ground ahead. Nearly there, it seemed that those stumps didn't look quite right, and looking down, the underbrush we were passing over was now invisible in the dark below. Then, in my dim headlamp beam, the tree we were tightrope-walking along seemed to be caught in the Y of a large tree far above the ground!! No telling how high!

We reversed our course, not walking but with hands and thighs hopping along that trunk, until we could again see the ground below us, and hop off. Worked our way through the wet young trees and underbrush to find our control, then looked up in darkness and marveled at my very unwise route choice.

YOUNGSTERS IN THE BACK YARD

"I hear some youngsters playing in the back yard," said Phillips, "Are they all yours?"

"Heavens, no," exclaimed Professor Rogainer, an eminent numbers theorist. My children are playing friends from three other families in the neighborhood, although our family happens to be the largest. The Whites have a smaller number of children, the Greens have a still smaller number, and the Black the smallest of all."

"How many children are there altogether?" asked Phillips.

"There are fewer than 18 children, and the product of the numbers in the families happens to be my house number, which you saw when you arrived," said Rogainer.

Phillips took a notebook and pencil from his pocket and started scribbling. A moment later he looked up and said, "I need more information. Is there more than one child in the Black family?"

As soon as Rogainer replied, Phillips smiled and correctly stated the number of children in each family. How many children belong to the Rogainers, the Whites, the Greens, and the Blacks?

The above problem, with some names changed, was offered to Neil Phillips during his trip to Washington State in late 1994. When given during the hike back from Boulder Cave to the parking lot, about 20 minutes over a rocky, rough trail on the Bald Mountain proposed rogaine map, Neil correctly solved it in his head without pencil and paper or hints.

Hint: You may find this table helps.

Rogainer	White	Green	Black	Sum	Product	Rogainer	White	Green	Black	Sum	Product
4	3	2	1	10	24	7	5	3	1	16	105
5	3	2	1	11	30	7	5	3	2	17	210
5	4	2	1	12	40	7	5	4	1	17	140
5	4	3	1	13	60	7	6	2	1	16	84
5	4	3	2	14	120	7	6	3	1	17	126
6	3	2	1	12	36	8	3	2	1	14	48
6	4	2	1	13	48	8	4	2	1	15	64
6	4	3	1	14	72	8	4	3	1	16	96
6	4	3	2	15	144	8	4	3	2	17	192
6	5	2	1	14	60	8	5	2	1	16	80
6	5	3	1	15	90	8	5	3	1	17	120
6	5	3	2	16	180	8	6	2	1	17	96
6	5	4	1	16	120	9	3	2	1	15	54
6	5	4	2	17	240	9	4	2	1	16	72
7	3	2	1	13	42	9	4	3	1	17	108
7	4	2	1	14	56	9	5	2	1	17	90
7	4	3	1	15	84	10	3	2	1	16	60
7	4	3	2	16	168	10	4	2	1	17	80
7	5	2	1	15	70	11	3	2	1	17	66

Answer on page 132.

SCIENCE OLYMPIAD – Where You Can Help Youngsters Get Involved in Navigation Sports

by Larry Berman and Bob Reddick

The Science Olympiad is a nationwide academic, interscholastic competition designed to increase student interest in science, and improve the quality of science education. There are about 32 individual and team events for which students prepare during the year. The annual competition tournament takes place during the school year at high school or college campuses, and has a format similar to game shows, TV shows, and the Olympic Games. Team effort and a cooperative group planning skills arc emphasized. Fields of biology, art, earth science, chemistry, physics, life sciences, ecology, and technology are the science disciplines involved. This article focuses on just the two events closely related to orienteering: Road Scholar and Nature Quest.

In February 1994, Bob Reddick was asked to assist the students in four teams to prepare for the Washington State Championship, in which 116 teams from middle, junior high, and high schools across the state would compete. These four teams had taken first through fourth place in the regional play-offs in December, and were getting ready for the state finals. The state finals were held in March, and two state teams went on to do well in the National Science Olympiad at the University of Arizona at Tucson, on May 21,1994.

Larry Berman has helped coach a local team for 4 years, first working with the Nature Quest team, and this year with the Road Scholar team.

The 10th National Science Olympiad Tournament takes place on May 20th, 1995, at Indiana University, Bloomington, IN. So to get the highest visibility for promoting the connection with orienteering, volunteers should offer themselves to the state championship team, for the period April to early May. But in any event, check with your local school to see if you can help their team. It involves a few hours teaching kids about maps and compasses. It is an opportunity to get your local event schedule into the hands of some of the brightest and most motivated students, and may even get you some new young members for your O-club.

The Nature Quest event is a combination of a scavenger hunt, orienteering, and nature study for teams of two. The course is essentially a regular, easy orienteering course, but with just written directions to each control, involving compass use. The controls are exhibits or natural objects about which questions are asked. Compass directions, pace counting, and speed are a part of the event—usually just 50 minutes to complete the course. Elapsed time in minutes is subtracted from the points given for correct answers to give the final score. The course cuts through campus buildings but remains on the campus grounds.

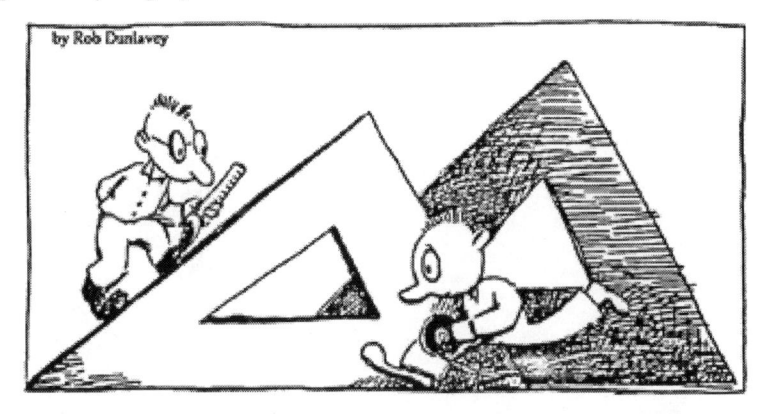

The regional and final state tournament locations are known in advance, so you can do some field work to prepare. I found that about half the students in the event had some familiarity with a compass, but did not know about magnetic declination, and had no practice in running a course, and no orienteering experience. To prepare for Nature Quest–the first effort should be to get each student a compass to use for

Published in the *Orienteering North America* February 1995 issue.

the entire preparation period. The simplest baseplate compass will do. Each student should have a chance to use the compass for several weeks in different surroundings. One practice exercise we used was from Kjellstrom's Be Expert with Map and Compass (page 75 on indoor practice). The game consists of hanging about 12 signs with numbers from 1 to 12 around a large room. Each sign has a corresponding numbered sign for the floor, placed on the opposite side of the room. Each student has a numbered card to record bearings on, with lines numbered from 1 to 12. The students take positions on their numbers around the room, sight on the wall sign opposite, and record the bearing. About each 30 seconds, the instructor says 'move', and they all move around to the next numbers. We collected the results, and at our next training session discussed the errors made and the accuracy of the good bearings. Most students, after just 5 minutes of instruction, were able to get about 8 of 12 bearings correct within 10 degrees. Common errors were the famous "180" (reading south for north on the needle), and misreading or miscopying the angle from the dial.

The next training to simulate the real event is to run a practice course or two on the school campus. The coach can furnish each student team of two a schoolground map, roughly drawn, plus a set of written directions. This is very similar to an orienteering description sheet. The event differs in that the control locations are not shown on the map, but are described in words with direction headings or bearing and distance directions. Example: 'Go out north door, turn West, go 150 meters, turn south and climb hill. What species of plant do you find at the top? (Write it down).'

The Road Scholar event is a map reading event, also about 50 minutes, with correct answers to road and topographic map questions determining the score. Teams of two work to read the state road map and one or more USGS topographic maps furnished to each team. The coach should try to obtain a campus map in advance for each venue where local, regional, and the national events will be held. Have the students do a table map exercise, following written directions around a simulated course the coach makes up for each location. The manual for the event includes exercises, and actually has last year's test, and these can be used as models.

The questions and area of interest are secret until the event starts. Students may use protractors, rulers, and calculators if needed. Questions involve map scale, legend, tables, locating symbols and features, taking bearings, interpreting contours, determining stream gradient and flow direction, land survey questions for the high school level teams.

Most states are involved in this worthwhile activity, and your local middle to high school science teacher can tell you if their school is entered, and if they need a volunteer coach.

SURVIVING YOUR FIRST ROGAINE – How to Do It Right the First Time

For orienteers who haven't yet participated in the long-distance version of the sport, here are the basics: A rogaine is a rugged, outdoor, group or team activity involving cross-country navigation and endurance. No, it's not an acronym. The name was coined from the names of the founders in Australia back in the 70's, with the first Victorian Rogaining Championships held in 1976. Your team of up to five members receives a USGS-type topographic map and a description sheet showing about 50 controls of various point values scattered over about 100 square kilometers of the venue. You have two hours to plan your likely route during your 12 or 24-hour event time. A mass start typically is at 12 Noon, and teams scatter in all directions. At about 6 PM a food tent opens at the central Hash House for continuous serving. The smart teams loop back there to eat, rest, refresh, and prepare for the remainder of the event. The finish is at 12 noon the next day, with more food and awards. Highly competitive teams will reach most of the controls; those out to enjoy some great scenery and some challenging navigation will "win" no matter how many controls they visit. So here is a checklist of sorts on how to make your first rogaine survivable AND enjoyable:

1. PARTNER. Find a compatible partner or partners. Will his/her fitness disappoint you, and hamper the team? Or vice versa? Will someone wimp out at night or get lured back to the Hash House with the thoughts of food and rest when you're five kilometers out and in an unexpected downpour? Ask yourself, "Why am I doing this?" Find a partner of similar mind, then "just do it."

2. FITNESS. Get mentally and physically prepared for the rogaine. Run or walk longer distances than you're normally comfortable with, while reading the topographic map of your practice area. Practice with your partner and your loaded fanny or day-pack and other gear. Try some night navigation. Fit your team's capabilities to your route selections. The best teams seem to find the routes that minimize both steep ascents and total climb.

3. GEAR. Carefully fit out your lightweight (10 pound) rogaine pack. Include the essentials (matches and lighter, knife, compass, emergency food, first aid kit, extra clothing, toiletries, pen and paper, I.D., flashlight and batteries, plus water, water treatment, and a whistle. Many take no sleeping gear, but you should take something for emergencies. Carbo-load before the event, and use energy foods during it. A new item being marketed is a tube of energy-drink-type carbohydrate pills that you can chew, instead of mixing gooky powder into your water supply.

4. PRACTICE. Yes, team practice, going up sleep slopes, in level but brushy terrain, and downhill, estimating your best and worst team speeds. Overall rates for the 12 or 24 hours will vary from 1.5 km/hr (KPH) to 4 KPH for the wide range of teams that compete. Predict your arrival time at easy-to-find features. If your actual time of arrival is within 10%, or +/- 10 minutes of your estimate, you're O.K. Assuming 48 or more controls, averaging 50 points per control, a world-class team will gain about 100 points per hour, or about two controls per hour. An average recreational team doing a 12-hour event will gather perhaps 12 controls and maybe 400 points. Set your goals high, but grin and accept what Mother Nature allows.

5. WATER. Estimate your water consumption rate. Food will matter little during the 24-hour event, but you can't go on without water. Carry three water bottles, drinking one per hour while moving. Drink about 16 ounces of a sports energy drink just before the event. You've drunk enough if you have to void a lot. Locate water refill sources on the map while you're planning your route. You can't leave

the slowest teammate behind, so keep all healthy—which means hydrated. Dehydration ruins your mental processes, too!

6. MEASURE. Time and pace-count on every chancy leg. If ail partners are pace-counting and timing each section from one prominent feature or attack point to the next, you won't get far off. As you might expect, this is surprisingly hard to keep doing over a 24-hour period. There will invariably be parts you blunder on–such as walking right by the not-obvious trail junction, and the missing the vague, nebulously set control in the dark. It's fun to share experiences after the event is over: The beginner team that took the bomb-proof route into a difficult control and nailed it in the dark, while the "'elite" team never found it in broad daylight–great sport!

7. LOST? You won't get lost if you always thumb your map—keeping track of just where you are at any time. Use both pace counting and timing to nail some easy intermediate points en route. When you forget, or didn't because the leg was "too easy," relocate to an identifiable rock-solid feature. Large or linear features are best. Plan for this "bail-out," and set a time limit of 10 minutes, after which you give up your aimless wanderings!

8. CHECKUPS. Frequently double-check your partner's condition, navigation, mood, and energy level. Revise your initial plan when things don't work out (they never quite do!). Late returning teams are penalized at 10 points per minute. With just one hour left, you should be within about 2 km of the Hash House finish, with just one control left to get.

9. NIGHT. Night navigation takes about the same application of skills as daytime. You want to be in the part of the map that is very open, or has a dense trail system, and many linear handrail features. Try to avoid sleep climbs and descents after dark, when footing can be critical. Headlamps often don't show all you need to maneuver well, so use a flashlight, too. It is somehow comforting to think (as you crash through wet brush in the dark) that seventy percent of the rogainers are back at the Hash House, digesting the great food you paid for, and curling up in cozy sleeping bags. Pitiful! Yes, they're losing points and missing out on the best part of the rogaine!

10. REST. Few rogainers can move for 24 hours continuously. Plan to rest and relax at water stops, try to swing back by the Hash House at mid-event, and always stop to treat any hints of blisters or injuries. Rogainers often are surprised to find that they achieve results far beyond their anticipated endurance capacities. But don't think you can "gut it out" without rest, water, or attention to your sore spots. Invariably your team will suffer the consequences if you try! To summarize, the old saying about "plan your work; work your plan" fits rogaining very well. Find that partner, get fit, select good equipment, practice, plan water use, time and pace-count, plan for relocation, check up on your partner, pick good night travel areas, and plan rests. Yes, just do it, but do it the way that will make your rogaining even more fun.

SHOCKING NEWS: True Origins of Rogaining Revealed!

It is generally believed that rogaining was originated in Australia back in the 1970's with the first Victorian Rogaining Championships held in 1976. These events, like the Bald Mountain Rogaine in Washington State, USA, coming up in August 1995, are generally 12- or 24-hour score courses covering 100 or so square kilometers of rugged terrain. You and your partner or team attempt to navigate to as many of the 50 or so controls as possible, using compasses and special topographic maps premarked with all the features you'll navigate to. For most participants, rogaines are a fun way to enjoy two day-hikes with a great campout and lots of good food and company in scenic surroundings. For others, they're the most challenging of ultra-marathons, with tough navigation and night orienteering thrown in.

But that widely held belief in the origin of rogaining has been shattered!! The world will be shocked to learn that rogaining, or "roganing" as it was called then, pre-dates the Aussie "invention" by two centuries! At least it appears that way, after you examine the following document recently located in another old British colony. It is printed here in full, as translated into more modern English. JUDGE FOR YOURSELF THE TRUE HISTORY OF THE SPORT. You may also find these old "orders" helpful right now in planning your participation in modern "rogaines."

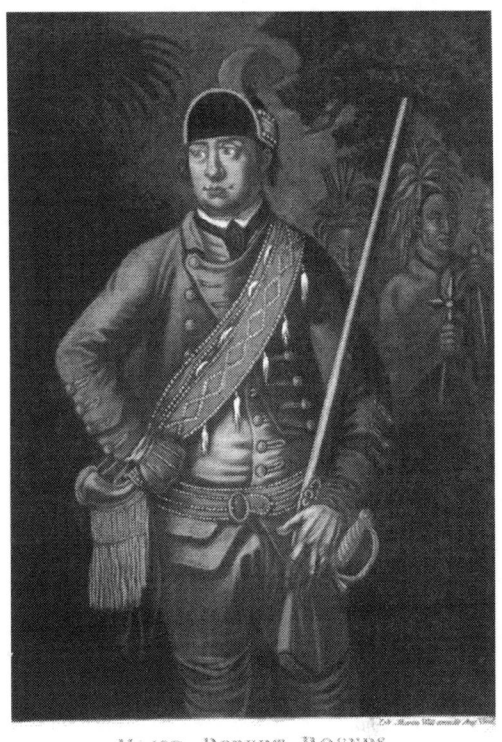

MAJOR ROBERT ROGERS,
Commander in Chief of the Indians in the Back Settlements of AMERICA

Standing Orders, Rogers' Rangers Roganing

by Major Robert Rogers, 1759*

1. Don't forget nothing.

2. Have your backpack with survival gear clean as a whistle, hatchet secured, trail food and three jugs of water, and be ready to march at the announced mass start time.

3. When you're on the march, act the way you would if you was sneaking up on a deer. See the wildlife and competing teams first, but don't let them distract you.

4. Tell the truth about what you see and what you do. There is a quest of roganers depending on us for correct information about our sport. You can lie all you please when you tell other folks about your rogan, but don't never lie to a roganer or an official.

5. Don't never take a chance you don't have to. Find the easy way around obstacles.

6. When we're on the march we march as a team, only so far apart at any time so's one can always see or hear the other teammates.

Published in the *Orienteering North America* July 1995 issue.

7. If we strike swamps, or soft ground, we go single file, and help each other to get safely through.
8. When we march, we keep moving even after dark, so as to give our competitors the least possible chance to outscore us.
9. When we camp, we eat and sleep fast, repair our wounds, and awake early to finish the course.
10. As we punch in at controls, we sign in on the intention sheets, so if we have any troubles the searchers can find us fast.
11. Don't ever march home to the Hash House the same way, take a different route so you'll find the most controls. Two or three big loops work jest fine.
12. No matter whether we travel in big parties of five, or little ones of two, each person has to keep watch ahead, to the flanks, and behind, measure & time distances, & read the map so the team can't be surprised & wiped out with overshooting, parallel errors, or other bad navigation.
13. Every night you'll plan where to go if you get tired, torches go out, blisters hurt too much, or hunger overcomes fun.
14. Don't sit down to eat anywhere near a control, and don't help other teams or lead them in or out of a location.
15. Don't sleep beyond Beginning Morning Nautical Twilight, or dawn at the latest. Dawn's when those other recreational teams who've rested get up, have a big breakfast, and start out again. Those fiercely-competitive teams didn't sleep but keep moving all night.
16. Don't cross a river unless really fordable. Find slow or shallow spots, then use a long stick to probe for holes and for a third leg for support. Sticks work good for climbing and descending steep spots, too.
17. If somebody's trailing you, make a circle, come back on your own tracks, and threaten to ambush the folks that aim to misuse your skillful navigation. Resist the temptation to waste them with your hatchet. Remember, scalping is no longer authorized!
18. Don't stand up when a competitive team is following you. Kneel down, lie down, hide behind a tree. If at night, light the way to the edge of the map then cut your lights and hide. They'll never get back once off the map.
19. Let the controls come to you as you navigate all the way, then finish them off with a punch in your control card. Do that enough times and you'll win!

*translated by Major Robert Reddick, ret., who made only minor casuistry revisions in the original text of Major Robert Rogers (1731-1795), an American frontiersman. I found that old handwriting really hard to read. I also found what looks like lines under some of the words: <u>RO</u>GERS R<u>AN</u>GERS STAND<u>ING</u> ORDERS. Seems he may have invented the sport called "roganing" back then!

ROGAINER ALMOST DOES LAST RELOCATION

On April 20, 1996, while spectating at the Navy Recreation Center 24-hour Eco-Challenge (hike-bike-canoe) event at Jim Creek, WA, I was walking down a forested spur by myself and suddenly encountered an acute incipient large anteroseptal infarction, later accompanied by five nasty little fibrillations—all of whom were extremely unfriendly!!! Let me assure you that I would much rather have met an angry Sasquatch face to face.

Just had time to dig out my orienteering whistle from my pack and signal for help. Thanks to God and a superbly organized and capable event support team, plus competitive team #5, within a very short time I was on a 14-footed litter going downhill to meet the just-arriving medivac van. Only took some clotbuster and five jumpstarts to get the old ticker going again, and then . . .

But enough of all that for now. On April 24th the experts diamond drilled me out, and I'm heading for home today. A lessons learned article is now in the works, for early publication in the *IRB*, *Bearing 315*, and *ONA* (yes, you're now warned).

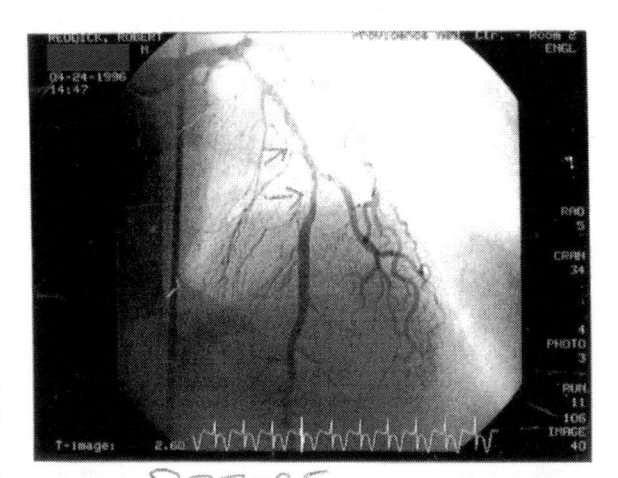

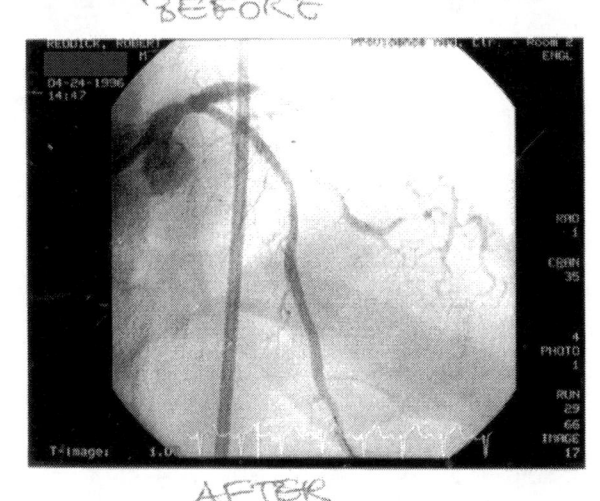

BEFORE

AFTER

Published in the *Bearing 315* May 1996 issue.

WHO OWNS THE AARDVARK?
Rogaining Puzzle for Those Temporally Unchallenged

There are five tents, each a different color and owned by rogainers of different nationalities, with different pets, drinks, and chewables.

- The Brit sleeps in the red tent.
- The Aussie owns the Doberman.
- Decaf coffee is drunk in the green tent.
- The Canuck drinks green tea.
- The green tent is just to your right of the white tent.
- The juicyfruit chewer owns the rattlesnake.
- Redhots are sucked on in the yellow tent.
- OJ is drunk in the middle tent.
- The Yank sleeps in the far left tent.
- The rogainer who blows bubblegum sleeps in the tent next to the rogainer with the coyote.
- Nonfat milk is drunk in the tent next to the tent where the donkey is kept.
- The Big Red chewer drinks rice wine.
- The Kiwi chews jerky.
- The Yank sleeps next to the blue tent.

SO, WHO OWNS THE AARDVARK?

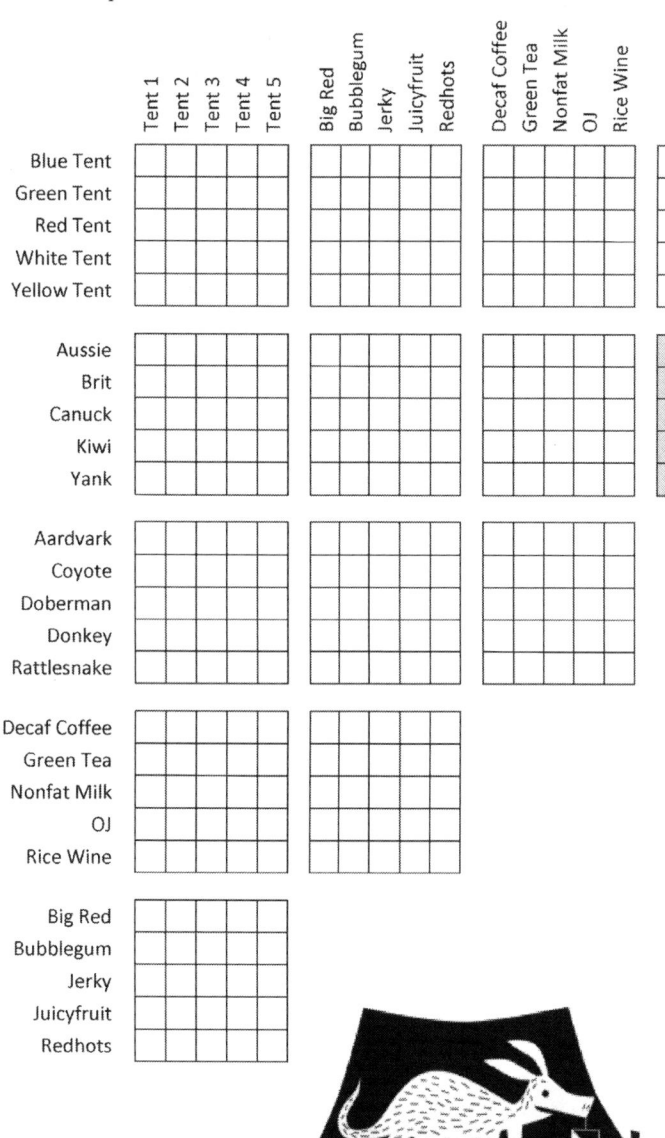

Solution on the copyright page.

Published in *Orienteering North America* August 1996 issue.

ARIZONA ROGAINE – North American Championships: March 1-2

A Rogaine is a very long distance, score-orienteering event, done by teams. Controls are scattered over a wide area, so wide that USGS maps are used instead of the usual O-maps. Generally, the maps are given to the teams an hour or so before the official start, so they can plan their route strategy: how to take the controls so as to maximize their point total. In North America, rogaines are done for 24 hours and fractions of 24, anywhere from 3 to 12 hours.

Quoting the event information by Wilkey Richardson: "The weather in Arizona around the first of March is usually sunny and mild. It is possible, however..." Ken Lew and I drove into the Empire Ranch meet area southeast of Tucson at about 11:30 PM on Friday night (Feb 28th) in a blinding snowstorm. Almost couldn't find the ranch road, in spite of detailed directions. Setting up a tent in the snow on a cow-pasture littered with snow-covered unknowns at midnight, then trying to sleep in subfreezing temperatures before the 10 AM start proved challenging. The North American Championships for rogaining (24 hours), plus 4, 8, and 12-hour events was well attended by 68 teams, with 148 competitors from Western and Eastern Canada, and throughout the U.S. Many ultra-marathon types, an Eco-Challenge team in training, and those us of just there for fun had a great time!

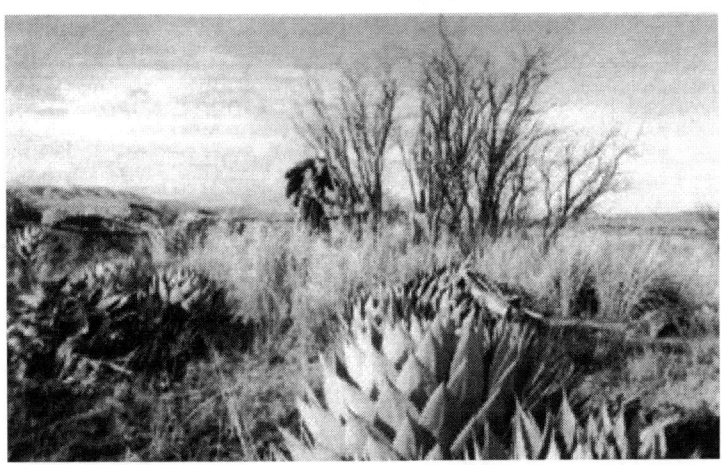

Ken Lew heads into the control, keeping the large Century Plant cacti at a distance.

By 11 AM on Saturday the weather had warmed, the sun came out, and the rest of the event was just about perfect—given the 4600+ ft. elevation and the dry desert air. Teams scattered in all directions from the base camp (Hash House) at the start time, going for scores at the 65 controls scattered over nearly 200 square km of former ranch country, now BLM land (US Bureau of Land Management). Controls were all well-sited, the map was excellent, and the navigation was generally easy. Lots and LOTS of barbed-wire fences made nice handrails, but slowed progress for those not able to leap over four feet with a pack on! Hostile plants were common, and sharp spines, some with sly hooks, awaited the unwary. Many birds, including hawks, some deer, and a herd of javelina (a wild boar), jackrabbits, bobcat tracks, and one black coyote were spotted. The Hale-Bopp comet delighted those tough or sleepless souls up at 5 AM on Sunday.

> 1997 North-American
> 24-Hour Rogaine Champions
> F21 Pam James (NS) & Catherine Hagen (BC) 2440/M21
> Tom Possert (OH) & Adrian Crane (CA) 3170
> M45 Peter Gagarin (MA) & Fred Pilon (MA) 3070
> Mxd Eric & Mary Smith (NY) 1940

The following are some detailed excerpts of several of the top teams from Clint Morse's rogaine calendar on the web.

Published in the *Orienteering North America* April 1997 issue.

PETER GAGARIN who teamed with Fred Pilon commented: "got 3070 points and 57 of 65 controls...ran about 33 km, walked about 80. Nine hours, 8 minutes and 56 km on first loop, stopped 72 minutes (at Hash House), 13 hours 32 minutes on second loop, over 9 hours in the dark. The map was by far the best we've had for a rogaine. It did make me wonder from time to time if that was to our advantage, since we have more experience than most on really lousy maps, but was still a joy to be on. #40. Headed into the control. Daylight was fading. Looking for some vegetation object, assuming it would stand out from a distance, and went just south of the control and on another couple hundred meters. No 'unique vegetation', no 40 points, moderate panic. But the topography seemed to say we had overshot to the left, so we made one dash back and found it. Turned out to be some cactus disguised as a bunch of big artichokes. (See photo). #36. (Sunday morning) Now just a matter of getting as many low-point controls as possible without getting in late...I thought we might be able to get 21, 22, and 27 and pushed the pace. Fred started calling me a sadist, but I didn't take it seriously because he wasn't really swearing a lot and falling down and looking pale and emptying his water bottles to lighten the load when there's still an hour to go—you know, the things he does when he's really tired—so he obviously had something in reserve."

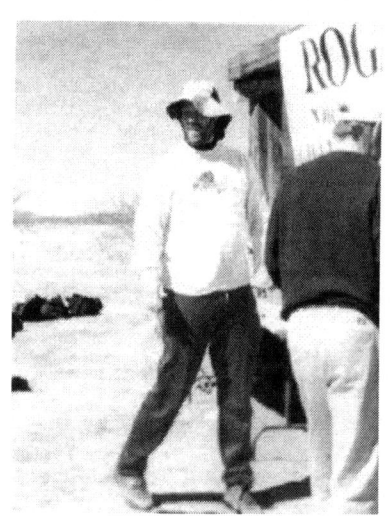

Wilkey Richardson, meet director (with floppy hat).

JEAN-JOSEPH COTE with Jim Baker: "Unfortunately, shortly after leaving #85, I brushed something with my foot that made a "brrrip!" sound, and a few seconds later I heard Jim cry out in pain, and he had just kicked the barrel cactus that I had brushed. It took the two of us a few minutes to get the thorn out of his shoe. I measured 75.7 km along our route, in 23:51 hours, with about 3.5 hours down time, and 36 controls."

CHARLIE DEWEESE with John Potter: "On the way to #84 we went along the wash, and thought that the fence that crossed the trail showed up much too early. We got distracted and spent 45 minutes combing the wrong wash system, before figuring out where we should be. Saw Stan Wagon and Cordon Hardman going the other way. Stan pointed out the bobcat tracks, and recommended control #88 as the prettiest placement he had ever seen. On to the muddy clearing at #48, slipped and fell in the ditch on the way out. (Later) we were pretty low, cold, and without food. On the way in we had our headlamps off, and saw two runners heading out with glow sticks dangling from their knees. They looked ridiculous, John thought they might be J-J and James Baker, but I thought this behavior was beyond even those two famous engineers. Found out later that it was indeed them. I think we ran about 74 km, collected 31 controls for 1870 points.'

STAN WAGON with Gordon Hardman: "We were the only team to go in shorts (we did use gaiters). Fine for the first 4 hours, but then there was a section of cat's claw cactus that ripped our legs up quite a bit. Two distinguished ultra-runners look first place, Tom Possert and Adrian Crane, with 3170 points and 61 controls. I was pleased that we nabbed the second veterans prize: we ultra-runners do very well in this sport."

ERIC SMITH with Mary Smith: "We set a reasonable route for ourselves in advance, did well on it in the daylight and rather poorly after dark, and ended up having to cut a lot of stuff at the end. 1:52 AM. Water at last. We had saved about half a liter of our original 2 liters, in case this (water point) was also empty, but it was quite a relief to be able to tank up. Getting quite cold by this time, and we had already stopped along the way to put on all the clothes we had and to eat a bit. The remaining water in our bottles was at this point already partially ice. Mixed up 1 package of ERG, filled the other bottles with just water.

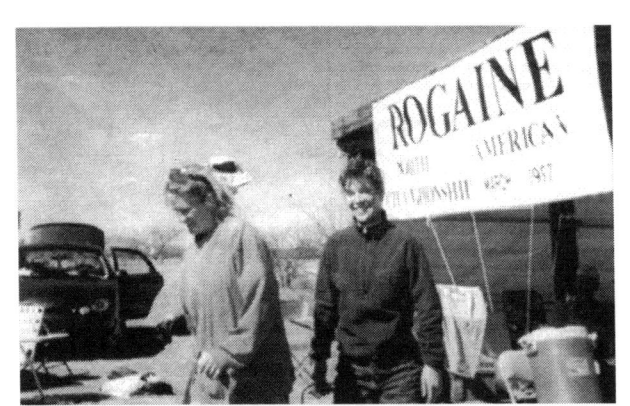

F21 winners: Pam James (Nova Scotia) and Catherine Hagen (British Columbia).

On leg to #54, followed fence line that had much more detail on it than shown on map, and we were beginning to really wonder where the heck we were getting to by the time the sun started lightening up the eastern horizon. However, the comet was really brilliant in the east on this leg, and that was an interesting distraction. Total points 1940, about 75 km, with 3 overshoots and mistakes."

ALLAN STRADESKI with Peter Mair: "Our first impressions of the rogaine site: This is a runners' course! Peter and I are not runners... Unlike most of the other teams, we planned a counter-clockwise route starting in the southwest. We felt that the handrails and greater contour information along the eastern and northern parts of the map would make for better night navigation. We would be more effective to get our limited running out of the way early by heading to what appeared to be the best running terrain in the SW quarter. We made good time and had picked up virtually all of the controls on the south half of the map by nightfall. While crossing through some of the tussocky ground between 40-64, I rolled my ankle bad enough that taping was required It provided a good opportunity to re-sock, refuel, and wade across the slough/creek. The presence of water in the wash also created a bit of anxiety in light of further planned crossings. We bare-footed it across going to #64. The total escapade, which included a snack and sock-change used up a precious hour of daylight. When the sun started to lower we also added a layer of Capilene (like polypropylene). Once across, our problems with this leg

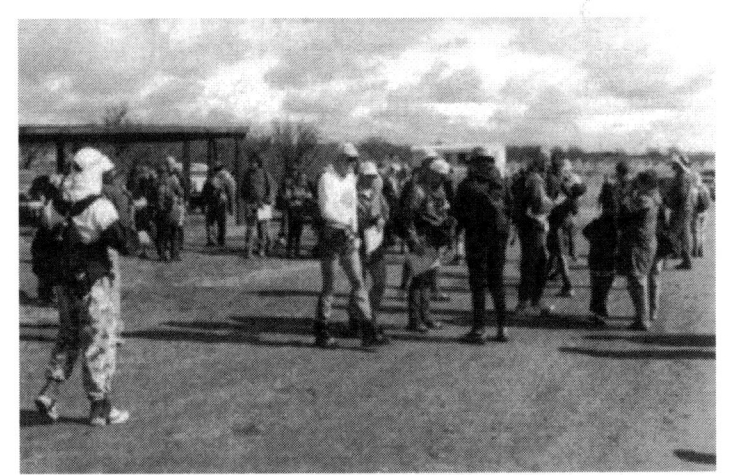

Starting the 24-hour event: in the center are Gordon Hardman and Stan Wagon, the only team to compete in shorts (and gaiters).

continued. Unmapped fences and marshes with water in them had us scratching our heads briefly. The fence line running south and the control finally led us in. 2950 points and 56 controls, about 102 km in about 21:45 hours. "

TOM POSSERT of the winning team carried, but did not use an Avocet altimeter, having not been told upon inquiry, that they were 'flat-out' illegal. For this event, it probably would not have helped anyway. Another minor variance: the teams coming in to the Hash House to eat or rest were not asked to turn in their control cards, which is a prescribed control measure by international standards. Tom liked the area, the lack of "fight", the great mapping, and the fact that event wrapped up with awards done by 11:15 AM on Sunday. He enjoys orienteering and the fun of competition, and thinks the 24-hour format is a real plus!

DONNA GOOKIN, partnering with Edwin, related that this was her sixth Arizona rogaine, her first in the 24-hour section. She had sworn she would never do long rogaines (the same as she had sworn about

109

marathons, but eventually did 40). The one inch of thick snow they encountered Saturday morning was a surprise, but they were pleased to see it gone by 11 AM. She heard about the comet, but was too tired at 3 AM to poke her head out of the tent to see it, (It was 29° F. at 5:12 am Sunday)

GAIL HANNA from San Diego O-Club, thought the course was very well planned, and after completing this 12-hour event, feels she'll be ready to do a 24-hour one. Her club is planning a rogaine ai Mt. Laguna soon. The Los Angeles OC also has one coming this year.

THE FOOD: Garry Cash did all the cooking for the event, running six propane double-burner stoves. The demand for hot water often outstripped the ability of the stove to heat enough, and the chili was cleaned out twice as fast as the vegetarian soup. Diane Ewald and Wilkey Richardson made the run in to Tucson to resupply the hot stuff for the carnivorous competitors. The spigot on the water barrel at the Hash House froze during the night, and the tiny campfire was really appreciated by the staff and those too cold to sleep.

A 6-MEMBER ECO-CHALLENGE TEAM-IN-TRAINING participated in the 24-hour, getting ready for the event next year in Queensland, Australia, Tom said they all were "having a good time", enjoyed the food, and found the people in the event all very helpful. He heard a pack of coyote near the herd of javelina they saw. The bigger boars were about 24 inches tall, with poor eyesight but a keen sense of smell, and very protective of their territory.

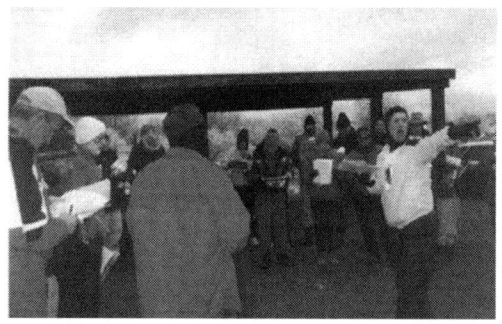

Mapper course setter Roger Sperline (on the right, pointing) gives the 24-hour starters final instructions.

BLAKE WOOD and Dave Scudder from New Mexico won the 12-hour. Blake has run two 6-hour rogaines at Los Alamos, and hopes to do more there. His team had "flamed out" near the end, started having night navigation problems, but really enjoyed the event.

VLAD GUSIATNIKOV with John Britton: Found shivering and with a bloody nose from hitting barbed wire, Vlad commented, "the night reflectors used at the controls could be better, but the map was wonderful and the event excellent overall. Best point-placement planning I've ever seen, with point values assigned very properly: an 80-pointer almost always was out of the way. Choice of control features could have been better, most of them too easy. A very appropriate overall size for an area and number of controls." (The overall winners got 61 of 65 controls, very near the 95% standard for an outstanding effort of an elite team in a given rogaine)

So the Arizona North American Champs are history. Now is the time to start YOUR preparation for the next NA Champs and the World Rogaining Champs (first time outside Australia) on August 4-5, 1998, near Kamloops, B.C. Canada. It's part of the Sage Stomp '98 extravaganza, for which see the homepage at oabc.bc.ca/ss98.htm.

And, good luck in the forest.

Route of Peter Gagarin & Fred Pilon, Winning M45 Team

We assumed that we could not get all the controls, and that affected our route right from the beginning. The basic plan was to do the NW section first, since we didn't want to be there at night; then the NE, leaving the center and SE for the night, and the SW for the final morning. It was hard to figure the best route, mainly because of the water stops. #60 was too far without water, #59 was out of the way, so we figured we had to go via #00, which meant that going 24-39-101-25-38-46-81-57-56 and then east along the top of the map would require a detour to 00. So we skipped 25 & 46 & got 81 on a dogleg (47-81-67). Then, #66, 84, 48. We went faster than we expected, reaching 48 in about 3.5 hours (vs. our expected 5 hours). After doing the NE section: #100, 104, 60, 89, 103, 47, 88, 68, 69, 65; we reached 65 in about 6 hours (vs. expected 8 hours). So, instead of the expected route straight back from 65 to eat and pick up our night gear, we had time for a bunch in the middle (33-59-30-26-85-45-64-40-29), hitting 29 with just a touch of light left in the sky.

Back at the finish after our really good first loop I still had my usual anxiety about the night. We did some good night orienteering, got lucky a couple of times, but should have taken direct routes more often: #102, 41, 23, 51, 82, 43, 63, 86, 53, 83, 55, 80, 54, 44, 52, 42, 32, doesn't seem to be well planned, since it crosses itself, but I'm not sure what is better. When we did try going cross-country (instead of along roads or fences), it worked fine, but we always felt that we shouldn't risk too much. Legs such as 23-51, 51-82, and 63-86 went fine on direct routes; we should have done the same on 53-83 and 42-32.

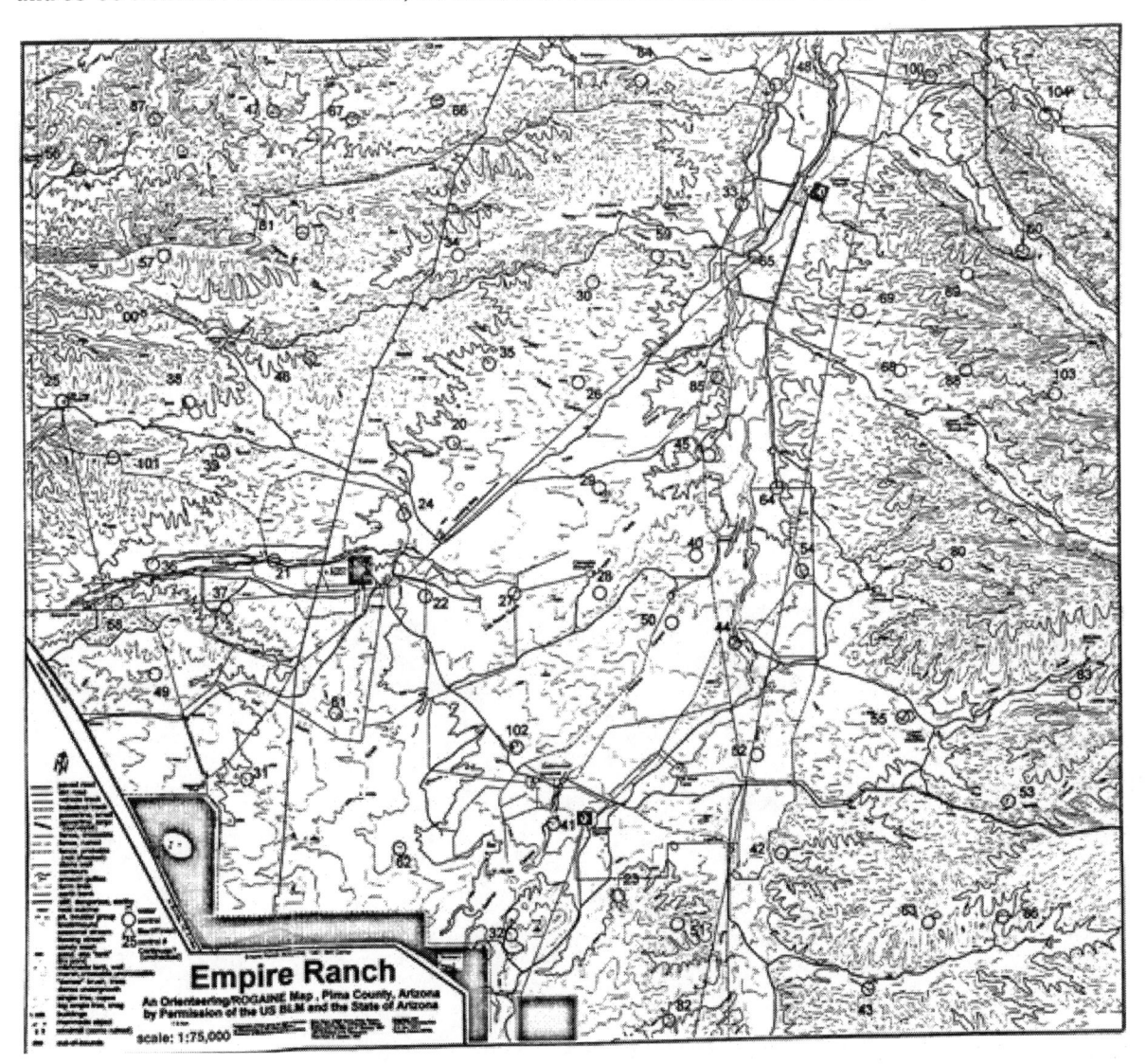

The final daylight part went well, almost all walking, as straight routes as possible: #62, 61, 31, 49, 36, 37, 21, 22, and finish.

Route of Allan Stradeski & Peter Mair, 2nd Men's Open Team

We felt that we should be able to get most, if not all of the controls, but we'd have to work hard. We planned to leave some of the lower pointers in the middle till last—if and when we had to bail out. Unlike most of the other teams, we planned a counter-clockwise route starling in the SW, to what appeared to be the best running terrain there. We felt that the handrails and greater contour information along the eastern and northern parts of the map would be better for night navigation. We made good time and had picked up virtually all of the controls on the south half of the map by nightfall: #24, 21, 37, 36, 58, 49, 31, 61, 62, 104, 41, 32, 23, 52, 42, 51, 82, 43, 63, 86, 53, 83, 55, 44, 50, 28, 40, 64, Cinco Windmill 54-80. While crossing through some of that tussocky ground between 40-64, I rolled my ankle bad enough to have to tape it.

We got off to a good start and had our best night ever: #103, 88, 68, 69, 89, 60, 104, 100, 84, 66, 67, 81, 47, 87, 56, 57, 00, Our plan provided the handrail/catching features which gave us good results. Our tapering food intake, however, caught up with us. By the time we hit #00 water station, we were running on vapors. Peter was getting quite cold despite wearing all clothing. We even considered heading home. Thank goodness for Power Gels. We really suffered timewise on this northern leg from poor energy management. We won't forget that leg for a while.

Early morning, we continued to pick up the points along our pre-determined route. We began to realize that some of the critical "biggies" back, towards the east would have to be abandoned: #25, 101, 38, 39, 46, 30, 26, 35, 20. The ridgeline was a "march to purgatory" (46-30), then we headed home, taking a few smaller morsels (controls) to finish off the 1997 North American Rogaine Championships. We finished with half an hour to spare.

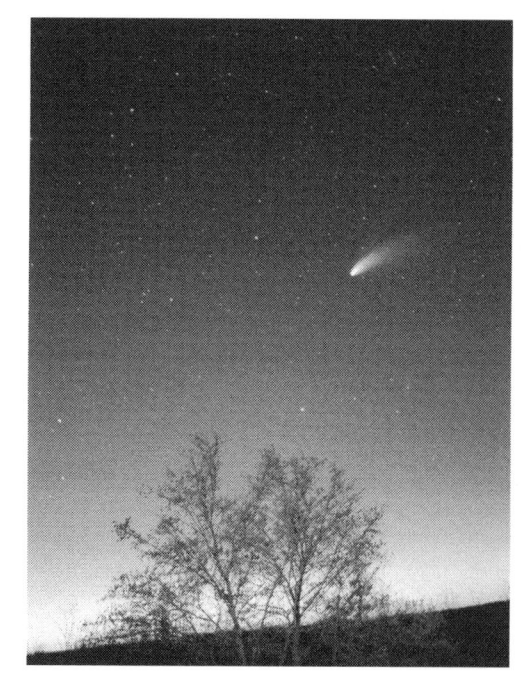

ROGAINE FOOD

Two old subjects came up this weekend while Les Stark and I were field checking the Takhlakh Rogaine map and proposed course. First, mysterious "gluttony factor", which always seems to surprise the most well-prepared rogaine organizer, who finds the abundance of food at the Hash House wiped out about 9 PM Saturday night! Second, the absence of any recent list of the basics in food and food preparation and serving equipment needed for, say 100 competitors at a 24-hour event.

Maybe a forthcoming book on the sport may address this, but it seems that this mail list is an ideal place to exchange successful lists, recipes, the favorite dishes that get consumed most rapidly, the most memorable dining experiences of rogainers over the years, etc. Even such niceties as an old-timer's recommendation that some of the key organizers could even spare a moment to personally deliver a hot plate of food to a team that comes staggering in late at night, and obviously barely able to even sit down!

And not to forget those whose competitive spirit precludes them from a HH visit until about 1 minute before time expires. What do they get, and do they deserve any priority in line (the queue), if any? And do we save anything for those not back in after an hour or so, or just presume them dead?

Should the most expensive/short supply items be rationed out? How about the smartest rogainers (arguably) who spent the bulk of their time eating, with some minor breaks for control finding? *[My favorite group, now.]* Are meal tickets used, or is everyone expected to pay the full fare for food, regardless if in 6, 8, 12, or 24 hour sections?

Any special requirements—such as food saved for the staff, vegetarian and other dietary needs (when known about)?

Has provisioning of water controls or surprise locations with fruit, juices, etc. been found practical, appreciated, etc. I've not seen or heard of this done except in Australia, but could be uninformed.

Why all this stuff on food? IMHO, great food/food service sticks in people's minds in relating positive memorable rogaining experiences, perhaps second only to 99.99% accurate control placement. (98% is a low standard around here!)

YOUR response is specifically solicited—please reply to all. Thanks.

Good Luck in the Forest.

Shopping List for Hungry Rogainers

Supplies for the Rogaine's 159 participants

Soda, assorted (64x12oz cans)

Coke (4 liters) (could have used more)

Snapple (48x16oz bottles)

Fruit Drinks (28x2 quarts) (tomato not popular)

Lemonade (5x2 gallons) (could have used more)

Gatorade (6x2 gallons) (mixed at half strength)

Swiss Miss hot chocolate (lots left over)

Milk, 2% (3 gallons)

Coffee (just a few servings used)

Tea (just a few bags used)

Bananas (60 lbs)

Oranges (30 lbs) (about 10 lbs left)

Apples (17x3 lb bags) (lots left, not popular)

Beef Patties (45 lbs, 4 patties/lb)

Veggie Burgers (5 lbs)

Hot Dogs (10 lbs all meat, 5 lbs chicken)

Hamburger rolls (160)

Hot dog rolls (160)

Published in the *Bearing 315* September/October 1997 issue.

Ketchup (2x40 oz)

Mustard (large bottle)

Relish (32 oz)

Cheese (5 lbs bulk, 3 lbs slices)

Bagels (14 dozen) (skip poppy seed next time)

Cream Cheese (5x8oz)

Slices Peaches (2x#10 can)

Apples Sauce (1x#10 can)

Fruit Cocktail (1x#10 can)

Baked Beans (1x#10 can) (not popular, some left over)

Chili (3x#10 can) (could have used more, including a meatless version)

Macaroni (10 lbs Rigatoni, 10 lbs elbows)

Spaghetti Sauce (4x#10 can)

Tomato Sauce (3x#10 can)

Canned Corn (1x#10 can)

Salt Potatoes (15 lbs)

Vegetable Oil for frying (a few oz)

Margarine (2 lbs)

Sugar (1 lb)

Salt and Pepper Shakers

Salt for cooking (1 box)

Pancake Mix (5 lbs) (more than enough)

Granola (4 lbs)

Instant Oatmeal (40 packets used)

Syrup (1x32 oz bottle)

Eggs (4½ dozen used)

Bacon (3 lbs)

Cookies (15 lbs)

Potato Chips (4 lbs)

Deli Salads (15 lbs each of 4 varieties)

Plastic bowls, styrofoam and paper cups, paper plates, plastic spoons, forks, knives (a few hundred of each)

Large Garbage Bags (20)

Charcoal (2 bags)

Propane, Gas grill with side burner, 2 burner propane stove, 3 bags of charcoal grill

10 cooler chests and ice for food

2 ice buckets for drinks

4x5-gallon coolers

5x55 gallon drums of water to supplement hand-pumped well on site

250 gallons water distributed at 5 water controls

WORLD MASTERS GAMES – How I Lost My Gold Medal

The 1998 World Masters Games, sponsored by Nike, provided competition in 25 different sports for people who qualify as masters in their sport of choice. The WMG were centered in Portland, OR. For orienteering, masters are 35+, with competition in 5-year age groups. Previous WMGs were in Toronto, 1985, Denmark, 1989, and Brisbane, 1994. These Games extended from August 9-22; the O-events from August 10-14. The Columbia River O-Club organized the O-competition, held near Portland and in Goldendale, WA. We plan to have an event report and results next issue, but here is a vignette from the WMG.

The Short Course Orienteering Championship, Tuesday August 11, 1998 started off roughly, with a start delay for maps, and the clear sky allowed the sun to build up a near-record temperature at Powell Butte. The Japanese contingent included Mr. Tadohiko Isogaya from Tokyo, who was shown on my start list (I was start chief) as an F70+ (female over 70 year old), but was actually an M80+ on Course 1. Among the other 44 starters was a write-in entry on my Course 3, a Mr. Udo Grady from British Columbia, Canada. His wife Ursula was pre-registered on this same course, and both I learned later had orienteered since 1960. He could have been an M65A, but I suspected he just might be my only competitor for the Gold in my M60B class.

Udo's late registration I learned about after the event. He was registered for discus, weight-throwing and pole-vaulting events for both weeks, and hadn't time for orienteering, although he'd competed with his wife in the World Rogaining Champs the prior week in B.C. But misfortune struck when his pole broke while competing, landing him on the edge of the pit and sending him to the hospital with a back injury. He'd been coached that week on how to bend his pole for more altitude, and had achieved three new personal bests in practice. His pole couldn't take a fourth bend, though. The doctor told him he was out of the meet, so he came to watch at his wife's event. He had secretly asked the Columbia River O-Club officials if he could enter with the proviso that if he did not medal, his wife would not ever learn of his entry. He was in!

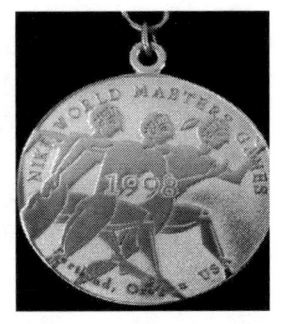

After all starters were away, I changed into my running (well, walking) gear for the hostile plant-filled fields and berry-vined terrain and was off on Course 3. At my third control area I encountered Isogaya-san, standing near a gigantic thicket bush—among several where my control stood hidden. I gestured to see if he was OK, since he'd been out about an hour on his shorter course. He nodded, and I saw that he was near a control, which proved not to be mine. Relocating quickly to a trail junction, I reattacked and punched in at my #3, then returned to the trail junction to head for #4. Isogaya-san came over and joined me, indicating some confusion. Without enough words in either language for us to communicate, we used lots of sign language. After checking his map, I pointed my route back to our common #3 several times to encourage him to proceed there, but he didn't move. Knowing that he'd win a medal to take home if he just finished his course within three hours, I couldn't leave him there. He then showed me his punch card, and the situation finally became clear to my somewhat addled and overheated brain. He'd already punched #3, but was stuck on how to proceed!

Mr. Isogaya's controls #4 and #5 were also the same as mine, so I pointed this out to him on my map and took off. He hung on my every step for the next two controls, with Jan Urban running to #4 just ahead of us, revealing the best route in through nasty vines. When #5 came in sight, I let him pass to punch and get water first. He looked at me with astonishment as I squirted water into the top of my hat, then he doffed his so I could repeat the treatment. While swigging from my Camelback bladder I checked his map.

Published in the *Orienteering North America* October 1998 issue.

His #6 control differed slightly from mine, so when we continued I gestured where he should diverge, but he hung on until his control was visible about 120 meters to the left of our route. To avoid further confusion, I punched my #6, then took a short break hiding in the shade of a tree until he continued on his own course. I nailed all my other controls, with only a major distraction approaching #9, when a berry-picker emerged from the bushes right in front of me. Funny how a teen-age, blond girl in shorts, plus a few almost-ripe berries, can distract from the total focus on navigation needed on this course.

So in to the finish, where I quickly learned that no one had yet seen or heard from Mr. Isogaya. I suggested a quick search, but just then he came in. I sure hope that I'm in as good a shape as he is if I reach his M80 class. (He took up the sport in 1986, one year before I did.)

Shortly thereafter, Knut Olson stopped to commiserate with me on my loss by less than a minute to Udo Grady for the Gold Medal! First I knew of it.

After the awards ceremony, hearing Udo enthuse over his award with his wife after being apparently shut out of the Games with an injury, I smiled. Udo went back the following week and competed in the discus throw, plus Silvered in the hammer throw. Mr. Isogaya got his Silver Medal, and when I received mine, we bowed to each other.

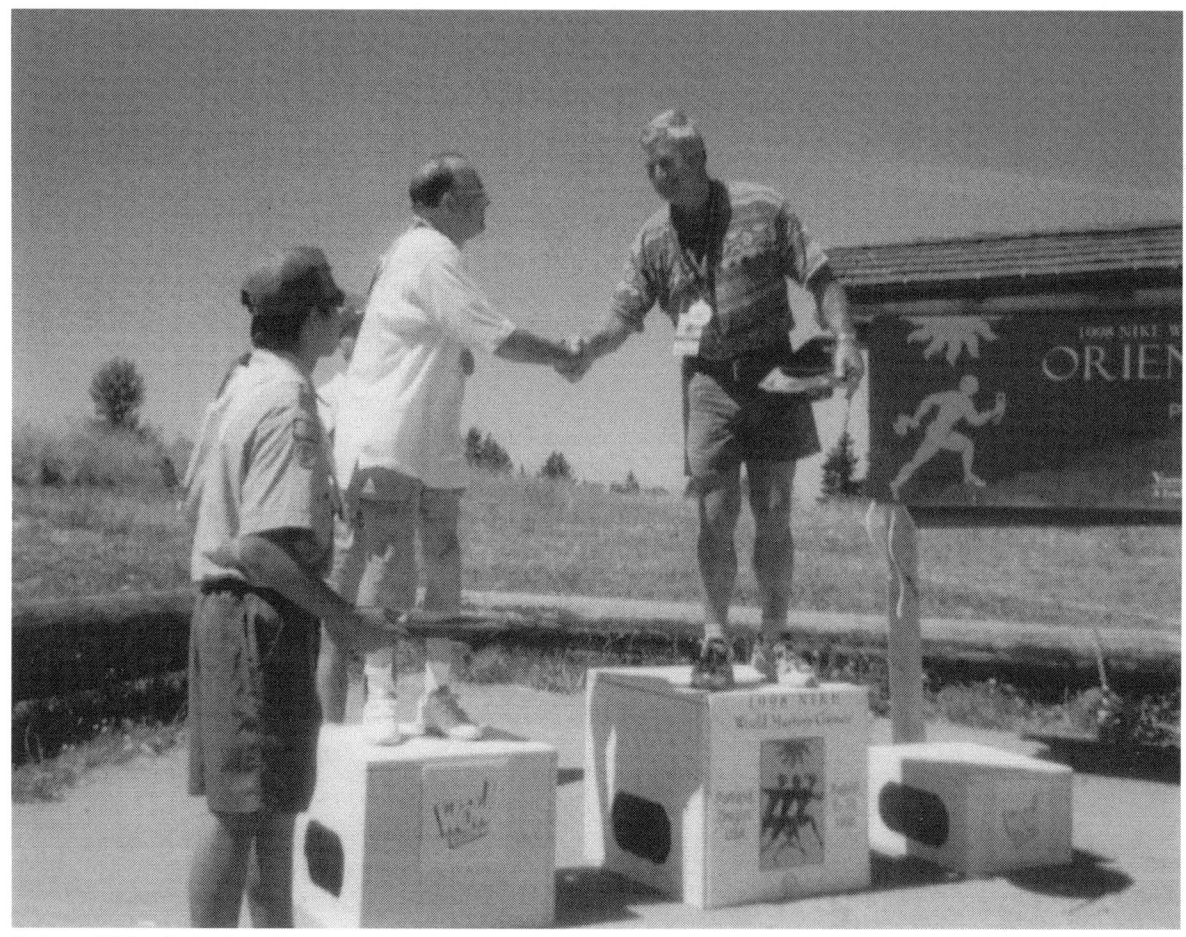

Bob and Udo shake hands.

1999 NOR-AM ROGAINE – Critique & Etc.

The sixth award for outstanding, meritorious service in the furtherance of world rogaining, Geoduck—*Panopea Abrupta*, was awarded to Michael Haynes of Halifax, Nova Scotia, organizer of the Maxi-Moose II North American Rogaine Champs, May 22-23.1999.

About the creature: The geoduck (pronounced gooey-duck) is found only on the Pacific coast of North America. Its name is derived from a Native American (Nisqually) word meaning "dig deep." These bivalve (two-shelled) mollusks bury themselves 2-3 feet below the sandy mud and gravel, using their long siphon, or feeding tube, to extract food from the water. Geoducks' shells average 5-8 inches, about half their body length, and add to their nearly 10 pounds. A geoduck can live to be 130 years old, living most of its life in one spot. Approximately 100 million geoducks live in the Northwestern coastlines.

The geoduck is also the mascot of Evergreen State College in Olympia, WA, and is sometimes called the State Bird! (Obscene references to its physical appearance are best left to the college crowd.)

Random comments on Nova Scotia and the rogaine: 170 participants—outstanding showing! Great support from the Amherst church group for food and conversation, the search and rescue folks who also competed, and the Scouts who tended a sleeping hut. Even parking attendants.

Results were published before Pat and I got home! Americans did quite well in all categories. Peter Gagarin and Ernst Linder once again did the impossible: captured all controls and got back early! Nice weather in Nova Scotia the whole time we were there, except for the Sat-Sun period. Competitors were thus saved from having to use sunblock, sunglasses, shorts, bug lotion, head-nets, excess drinking water, and seeking shady resting points. One black fly, however, seeing my guard down, bit me on the eyelid. Some competitors thought that mapping inadequacies should have argued against some control placements, but all controls were visited by a least one-third of the teams, so diligent navigating using all the terrain clues got results.

The organizers got lots of feedback on need for reflector tape on controls. (I'll get more detailed cost and source info together from 3M for reference soon.)

Since tourist attractions seem to open after June 1st (some at the end of June), in Nova Scotia—sunshine being one of them, perhaps the full moon dates in late June. July, and August should be given priority for Maxi-Moose III.

Pat and I had very good visits to the Maritime Museum and the Citadel (3+ hours) in Halifax after the event. The park staff told us the "those people on the third floor don't work on holidays", so we didn't get to see Andrea on Victoria Day. Enjoyed the Noon gun and 21-gun salute firing drills. Noted that Canadian reserve army artillery unit has females in gun crews. (Also advised staff that several display lights were out in the many historical displays and movie theaters, all of which were very well done.)

Put about 2400 km on our rental car, trying to do three provinces in three days! Got to the Anne Murray Museum. Fundy Fossil Museum at Parrsboro, Industry and Science Museum at Stellarton. Train Station museums at Antigonish. Kensington, and Tatamagouche, fossil digs at Arisaig Provincial Park, lobster tank at McKelvie's restaurant, ferry and longest bridge in world at Prince Edward Island, Anne of Green Gables historical site, old waterfront at Charlottetown, and slept in a 1911 caboose. Great trip! Too bad we were beaten out by two 19-year-old local males for first in our section, but in reviewing event I see that it was solely due to my parallel error for an hour on our second control!

Bob Reddick lives in Kenmore. WA. is a member of Sammamish O-Club, and has taken part in Rogaines since they developed in the US.

ELKHORN ROGAINE = CHALLENGING TERRAIN

Kittitas County, Washington has been the venue for three rogaines to date, the one at Buck Meadows in 1989, which was the first rogaine in the United States, the rogaine at Table Mountain in 1993, and the just-competed Elkhorn Rogaine. Rogainers find this is an ideal area to compete in, with comparatively low rainfall, open forests and sagebrush, and often-clear skies for moonlight navigation. Our rogaine on September 9-10 was just beyond reach of four big rainstorms that hit the Cascades during the event. Overcast skies, however, limited the almost full moon to about 10 minutes of illumination in our area. Some rogainers were navigating in a low cloud that blanketed the ridgeline to the south of the Hash House on Sunday—a new experience for them.

Sammamish Orienteering Club started the planning for this event about a year in advance—first getting the acceptance of Gene Martin, the ranch owner, to use his 18 square miles of land as the center of the needed 40 square miles for the course. Numerous visits allowed us to figure out the drivable road net, the ownership of private lands, and the willingness of owners to have us tramping over their property. We eliminated early on the northwest area, where owners were sometimes bothered by hunters, bikers, vandals, and other problems. One owner was reportedly in jail for burning his ex-wife's house down. We moved proposed controls off his land! During our field visits we encountered many of the 550 head of cattle, plus several herds of elk and a few deer. Jackrabbits, one snake, and many chipmunks kept out of our way, as did the five or so cougar known to be around.

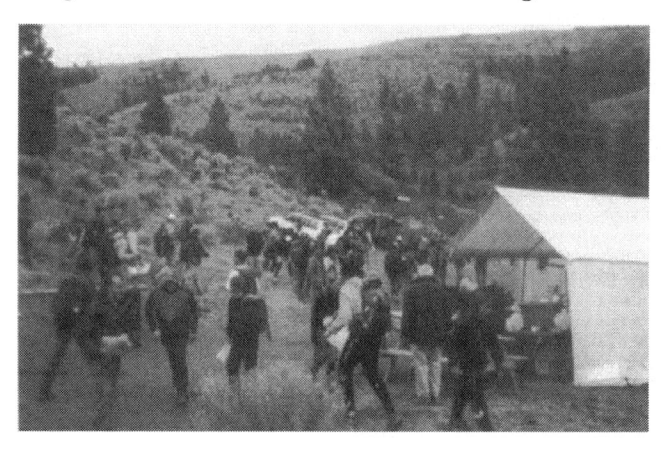

Sites Along the Course

An historic spot some teams saw was an original cabin used as a waystop on the old pony express route from Quincy to Yakima. Everyone hiked through the former main cattle drive route from Canada to the Columbia River. Competitors found the control sites fairly easy to find, even at night. But the ground in many areas was very rocky, and lots of steep hill-climbing was unavoidable. The overall winners, Eric Bone and Vlad Gusiatnikov, traveled an estimated 71 km in 21.5 hours, getting all the controls.

And They're Off

The 32 teams set out in several directions from the 10 a.m. mass start, with most heading for the northeast forested area, where many lower-score controls were located. Course Setter Dave Enger had carefully balanced the 52 controls so that roughly equal point scores would be obtained no matter which area was visited.

A lot of close-in controls were set for the 8-hour teams, and to help beginners get a quick feel for the map. Only two controls gave problems: 1) Control #41 was blown away by high winds sometime before the event, and was replaced when reported by an early-returning team 2) The other control, #68, deserves a compete story, for lessons learned for future rogaines.

Published in the *Orienteering North America* November 2000 issue.

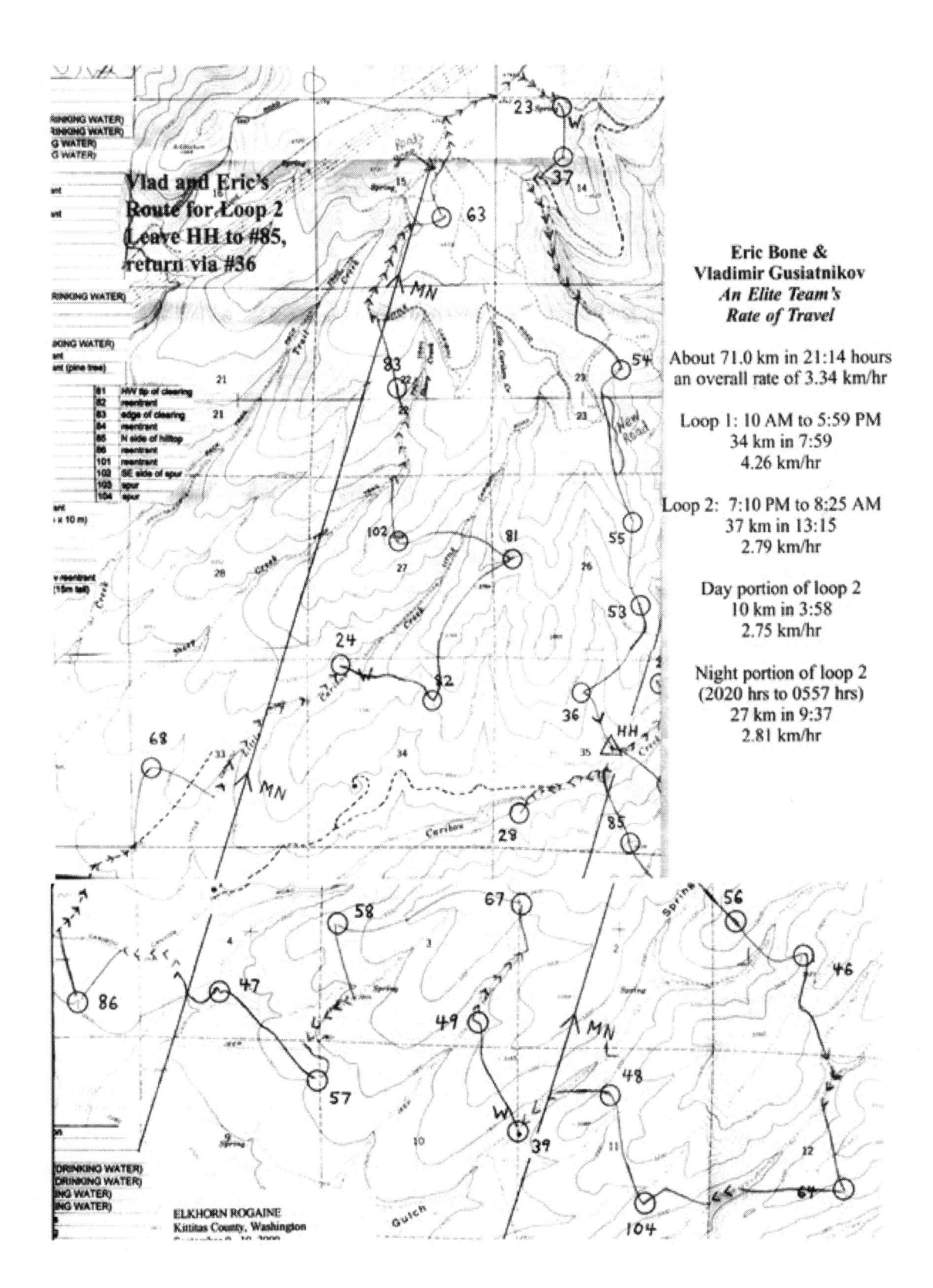

Vlad and Eric's Route for Loop 2
Leave HH to #85, return via #36

Eric Bone & Vladimir Gusiatnikov
An Elite Team's Rate of Travel

About 71.0 km in 21:14 hours
an overall rate of 3.34 km/hr

Loop 1: 10 AM to 5:59 PM
34 km in 7:59
4.26 km/hr

Loop 2: 7:10 PM to 8:25 AM
37 km in 13:15
2.79 km/hr

Day portion of loop 2
10 km in 3:58
2.75 km/hr

Night portion of loop 2
(2020 hrs to 0557 hrs)
27 km in 9:37
2.81 km/hr

ELKHORN ROGAINE
Kittitas County, Washington

The Story of the Mis-Set Control Number 68

In his original course design, Dave circled a point on a reentrant with a dry creek in the western part of the Elkhorn Ranch, where a section line likely to have a fenceline crossed the reentrant.

In April, I hiked in from the East about 800 meters from the Little Caribou Road (a jeep trail) to flag the proposed point with engineer tape. We flagged all the points early, intending that each of the some 50+ controls would be visited over several months by a flagger, a setter, and a vetter to independently verify it. These visits would also verify the accuracy or allow updating of the map in the area, spot safety hazards, and try to determine feasibility of night navigation to the points.

We also made minor additions to the USGS maps where we found new roads and buildings. We planned six water controls, actually had seven, with about 17 gallons of water at each. Actual use, on a cool and cloudy day, was only about one-third of that. Next time I would plan only 10 gallons each at just four water controls, assuming 80 or less people,

I pace-counted in on a compass bearing, crossed a newer jeep trail on top of the spur, and found only a faint sign of a removed fence-line running true north at the desired point, with no distinctive feature there. I decided to pace-count up the reentrant to a visible tall pine tree, about where the reentrant made a bend, and flag the tree with tape. When I returned home, I called Dave and told him to move the control circle on his master map the 150 meters I'd paced, and add the tree (50 feet, or 15 meters tall) to the description.

On another day, I drove up the new road from the ranch cabins which passed sites for new cabins, went to the section corner where two fences crossed, and recorded that the road continued as a jeep trail up the spur. I was puzzled to see a fence marching northward

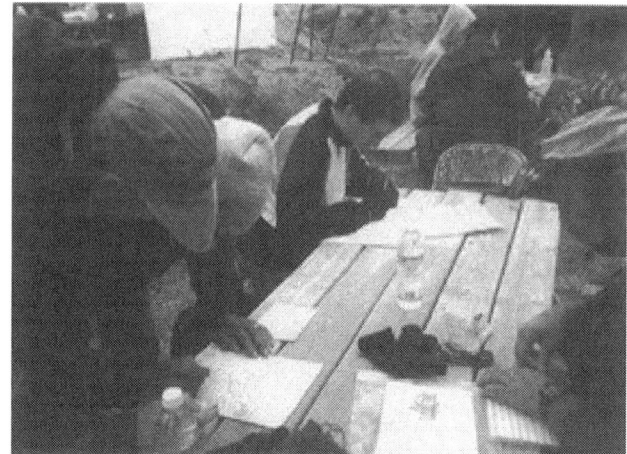

Vlad (hatless, at end of table) said he thought the course was well designed, since it took him about 40 minutes to plan their route. Normally, he said, this critical part of the rogaine takes only about 20 minutes.

from this corner, and wondered where it quit, since I hadn't seen it on my earlier visit to the reentrant. I didn't have time then to resolve the question.

On September 3, Bruce confirmed the location, saying that perhaps the tree was perhaps a little off to the northeast of his sighting. Two other similar pine trees were spaced about 200 meters apart up the reentrant, offering potential parallel errors.

On September 8, Bruce drove his two Czech Republic orienteer visitors, Ondrej Kotecky and Michaela Mahdalova, to that section corner, and they set off along that fence line to the reentrant (yes, it existed there), turned east and went the 150 meters to the mapped control circle. They found no pine tree there, so hung the marker and intention sheet for #68 on a short stump in a brushy tree area, clearly within the mapped control circle. They told Bruce, who later told me, that they didn't find the pine tree. This should have been a big warning signal that another visit, a map change, or a control description change should have been done. But the press of other last-minute business caused this to be missed.

During the rogaine, only six of 32 teams visited Control #68, including two at night. Their routes were up or down the reentrant, so the mistake had no impact on them. But one experienced team, Al Smith and Sharon Crawford, found the pine tree with flagging tape still in place, and then checked out the other similar tall trees with some loss of time. They were given credit for their visit there. Ken Lew retrieved the control after the event, taking the same route as the Czechs, and found the tree was some 200 meters beyond the mapped location. It's now clear that my first visit there was the root cause of the error, due to short pace-counting over rough rocky ground.

Course Planning

The procedure for flagging checking, vetting, and hanging control bags and intention sheets for rogaines is obviously very labor-intensive, requiring good navigators, good record-keeping, and some luck to ensure success.

I suggest for rogaine course planners that they carefully balance the overall course design with an eye toward economy of effort, by limiting the number of controls to somewhere in the range of 40 to 46 for a 24-hour event. Controls should be at least 1 km. apart, but not over 4 km, averaging about 2 km.

A circle of controls should be set around the Hash House to disperse the teams at the start. Total optimum length for all controls should be between 80 and 100 km, depending upon ruggedness of the terrain. The Elkhorn course had plenty of climb and rocky ground, but was only about 71 km. So the winning team, Eric and Vlad, had time for an hour's dinner break on Saturday, and wrapped up the whole course on Sunday 1 1/2 hours early!

VERGILLO, GROFF CLEAN THE MAP AT FIRST US METROGAINE, Held in Bremerton, WA

by Terry Farrah

Veteran rogaine organizer, Bob Reddick, thought he'd designed a course where no team would get all the controls. Reddick was way wrong. Team Magnetic Duo, comprising novice rogainers Dean Vergillo and Eugen Groff of Cascade OC, cleaned the map with more than an hour to spare at the Bremerton Metrogaine on Saturday, April 26.

"As soon as I knew Dean was to be my teammate it was unspokenly clear that a tough and very competitive race lay ahead of me," says Eugen Groff, originally from Switzerland and an orienteer since 1971, "He is a strong and fast long distance runner, and 15 years younger than I am. We decided to shoot for all the controls. We never doubted that we would be able to make it."

First US Metrogaine

A metrogaine is a long (typically 5-8 hours) team event with a Score O format: teams visit point-valued controls in any order, attempting to maximize their score within the time limit. Metrogaines originated in Australia and are quite popular there.

At this, the first metrogaine in the U.S., forty controls with a total point value of 2000 were located in and around Bremerton, a navy town on the west side of Puget Sound from Seattle. Fifteen teams gathered near the U.S. Navy destroyer Turner Joy on a temperate, overcast morning, for the 10:30 mass start.

Urban vs. Wilderness

Instead of punching in at each control, participants answered a multiple choice question about the control location.

For example, at the control pictured at the right, the question was: "By the guns the name in italics is (a) Hal, (b) Fletch, (c) Al," referring to a nearby plaque. Control 101 involved the team listening to a player piano and writing down the name of the tune, Those who didn't recognize the old song could instead write where the piano was made.

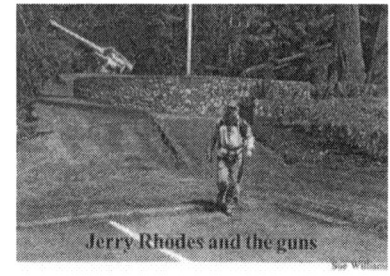

How did the metrogaine experience compare to that of a classic wilderness rogaine? "I'm kind of a snob about rogaines," says Curtis Condon of the fourth place mixed team, Beauty and the Beast. "How tough could it be to get a street map and run from control to control? But it's actually more difficult to find the control features because there's all this stuff going on. A manhole cover or plaque doesn't stick out at you the way a boulder or stream does." Condon would have run right past control 56, a plaque nearly flush with the ground, if his teammate, novice rogainer Miriam Condon, hadn't spotted it.

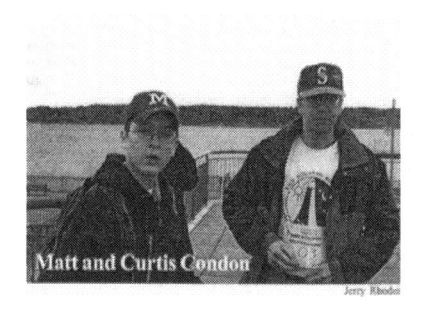

Beauty and the Beast was the top finishing team of three or more, and also the top finishing team with a junior member: 13 year old Matt Condon.

"Another neat challenge was the timing with the bus and the ferry," says the elder Condon. A single bus trip was allowed anytime during the race, and three controls in Port Orchard required a ferry trip.

"I figured the smart teams would go directly from the 10:30 a.m. start to get the 10:45 ferry," says Reddick. "So I went over to the dock with my video camera to check out this crowd. I got there and there was nobody." Bob just had to wait a little longer. Four teams did choose to take that first ferry, but they used their 15 minutes to snag up to three other controls first.

The bus option was offered because people might be tempted to take the bus even if it weren't legal. Many top teams did not use the bus. "We wanted to do everything on- foot," says Groff. "Also, we didn't think a bus ride could really shorten our running distance. And buses tend to be delayed regularly."

To minimize this uncertainty, and also to let the bus do much of the climb, several teams got on a bus immediately after taking the ferry back from Port Orchard. A drawback of this plan was noted by one participant: "It was an hour into the event and we'd already used the two things that could give us rest."

Five teams skipped the ferry jaunt. Because of the ferry schedule, it was not possible to spend less than an hour obtaining the 210 points in Port Orchard. "We averaged 238 points per hour on the mainland," says David Rogers, "so it wouldn't have been worth it to take the ferry."

Top Teams

"These were two hard chargers." Reddick says of top team Magnetic Duo. "really remarkable. Vergillo had been orienteering for less than a year. Groff said Vergillo was dragging him around the whole time. They ran the whole thing, finished at 3:22 p.m., and didn't even look tired."

The distance required to get all controls was about 24 miles.

Finishing second overall, and first for a mixed team, were Jonathan and Tori Campbell, also of Cascade OC and also novice rogainers.

"At the four hour point we looked at each other and said, 'This has ceased to be fun, what were we thinking?'" says Tori. "We kept going. We're gluttons for punishment."

The Campbells scored 1930, omitting only two controls.

"Every time I saw Jon and Tori they looked pretty intense," says Eric Bone, Jonathan's old college rival. Bone's team came in just behind the Campbells with 1750 points. Eric and his teammate, brother Nic Bone, walked the whole way.

"Eric was the packhorse, carrying all the food and water," says Nic. "The highlight of the day was about a third of the way through; it was sunny and we were on pace and I could still move my legs without pain. We kept ourselves in good spirits by discussing regular expressions and finite automata. I had significant trouble walking for several days following the event."

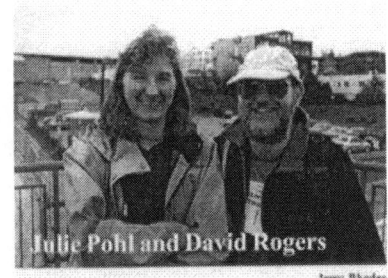

Julie Pohl and David Rogers
Jerry Rhodes

The Bones guessed the answers for the five controls they didn't visit, and got one right. "Considering there was no penalty for wrong answers it would have been foolish not to guess," explains Nic. Reddick's reaction: "I recommend future metrogaine organizers specifically prohibit guessing to prevent teams getting decent scores by remaining at the event center, scarfing up all the food, enjoying a quiet, restful afternoon/evening, and just filling in the score card with guesses."

David Rogers and Julie Pohl, a veteran (age 40+) team, managed to place fifth overall with 1430 points. This was the third rogaine for Rogers and the fourth for Pohl.

Recreational Division

Five of the teams entered the recreational division which allowed all forms of unmotorized transport. Dave Enger did the course on his bike and got all the controls in about five hours. Enger's route was similar to that of the Magnetic Duo, though in the reverse direction.

Two teams of local boy scouts also participated recreationally. Eric Brown, of team Penguins, got the idea from a fellow scout that the event would be a stroll around town. "The day of the race I saw the other teams synchronizing their watches, looking at their compasses and taking bearings, and I thought, 'Whoa, this is a lot more serious than just walking all around Bremerton.'"

Local Knowledge

For Bremerton natives, the race was an eye opener about their home town.

"It was always pointing out things that I'd never really taken notice to. 'What is the name of this field?' I looked at the map, I knew I'd seen it hundreds of times, but I didn't know its name," says Brown, referring to a field on his high school campus.

"I saw more of Bremerton than I ever wanted to see," says Sue Williams of Columbia River OC. Sue was born in Bremerton Navy hospital but lived there only a month or two. The metrogaine was her second orienteering event of any kind, and the first time she'd walked more than 10 kilometers. The metrogaine gave her an opportunity to get new landscaping ideas from the neighborhoods along the route.

"There were some really nice views, too," she says.

Asked for the highlight and the low point of their experience, Rogers and Pohl replied, "we learned never to ask natives for directions." Asking for directions was allowed by the rules. Rogers and Pohl asked a cab driver for directions to Coontz Jr. High School, near control 42. "He had an idea where it had been, but he directed us to a place nowhere near where it actually had been located. We immediately decided to proceed on our own."

Because the map was old (a combination of two 1952 USGS topo maps last updated in 1978, with minimal corrections), there were landmarks on the map that no longer existed.

Was this a highlight or a low point? "It's kind of low when you don't know where you are and a native who's supposed to know the town gives you directions that tell you to go way over there. Finding yourself is the high point."

Heather Clarke's highlight was a special tour of the Port Orchard ferry Carlisle II. She and teammate John Lee "were poking around downstairs where there's a little bar with a couple of taps. John asked one of the guys if they used it for parties. He said, 'You want to see something else cool?' He took us around and we got to do the rest of the trip on the bridge with the captain."

Finish and Future

Over the course of the event, overcast skies gradually yielded to sunshine for the finish at Evergreen Park, where everyone was served pizza. Reddick had polled the group before the start regarding what beverages they wanted, so everyone had their choice available. Everyone received a little wooden koala and a draw prize.

"We had so much fun," said Pohl, echoing the sentiments of many. "The town was about perfect with its combination of hills, parks, business and residential areas. Such a nice mix of urban scenery."

Although the event was sponsored by the Sammamish Orienteering Club, the Bremerton High School Naval Junior ROTC did much of the course development and provided the day-of-event staffing. Cascade members Heidi Bohn and Bill Cusworth vetted the course, yielding several corrections and improvements.

Will Reddick do this again next year? "Let's see how the Seattle event goes," he says, referring to July's Seattle Night & Day Navigation Challenge. "Sammamish will probably do another metrogaine. Meanwhile, I will be lobbying for other clubs to do these nationwide."

Orienteering Louisville is planning a 3-hour street-O for July 19, when it will be too hot, humid, and buggy to be out in the woods. At press time, Reddick was already trying to talk them into making it a full-fledged 6-hour metrogaine.

(A full-color complete map can be found at http://www.xoc.net/downloads/metrogaine.pdf)

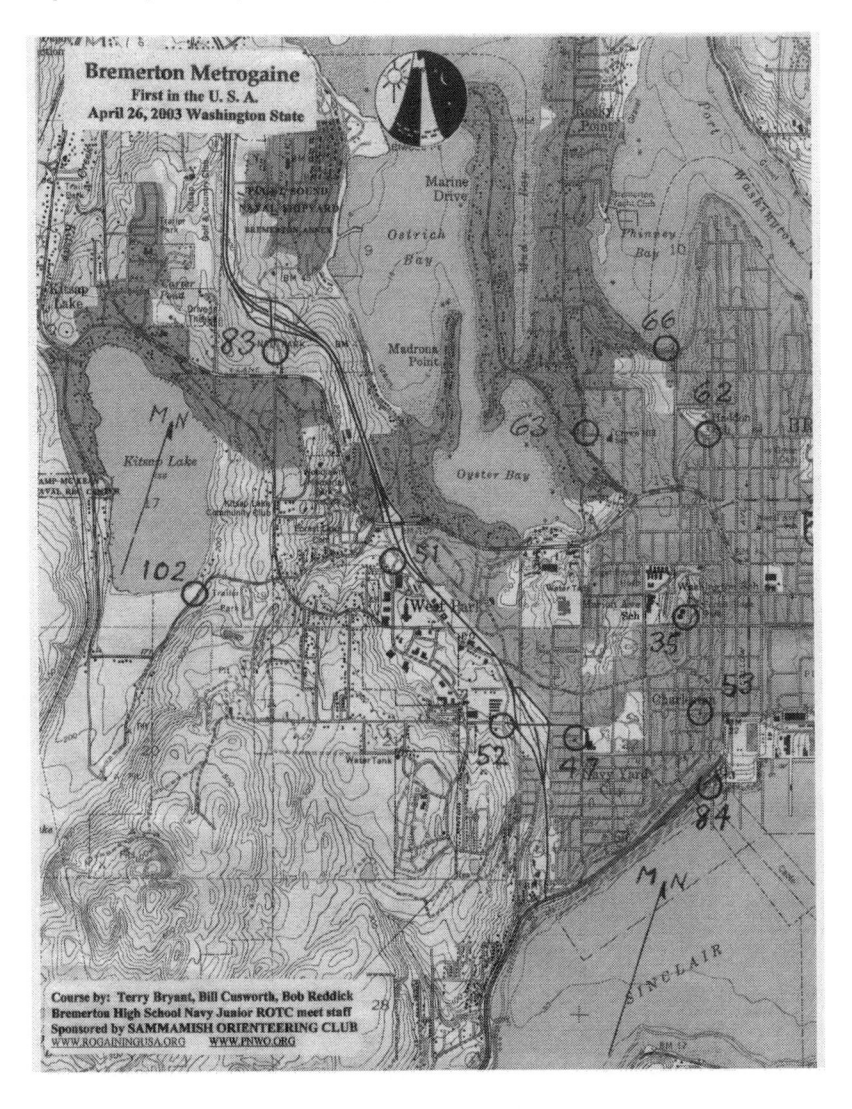

Neil and Rod Phillips Awarded Medal of the Order of Australia

On the Queen's Birthday on June 11, 2018, both Rod and Neil Phillips were awarded the Medal of the Order of Australia. The Order of Australia recognizes Australians who have demonstrated outstanding service or exceptional achievement.

Professor Geoffrey Neil PHILLIPS, for service to rogaining, to minerals exploration, and to education.

Dr Roderic John PHILLIPS, for service to rogaining, and to paediatric dermatology.

Bob Reddick wrote letters of nomination for each of them.

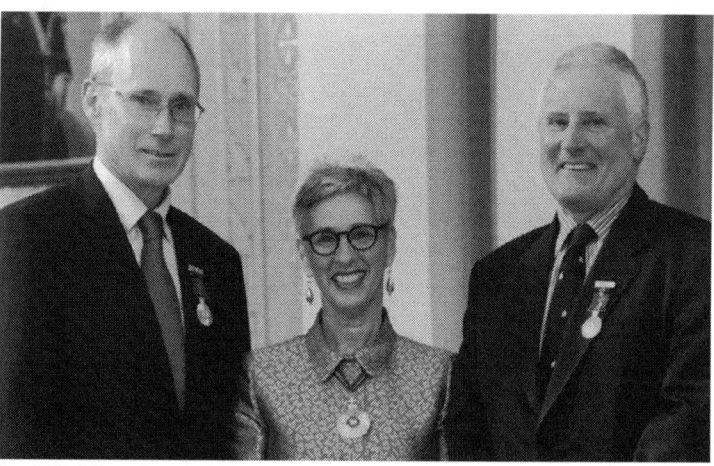

Rod Phillips, Linda Dessau (Governor of Victoria, Australia), and Neil Phillips

FIGMENT?

Bigfoot
Very hairy
Very scary
Nocturnal, foraging, cruddy
Endangered, maybe fictitious buddy
Sasquatch

by Rob Dunlavey

A poem to meet final requirement for my Junior Ranger Badge at Denali National Park, Alaska in August, 2018.

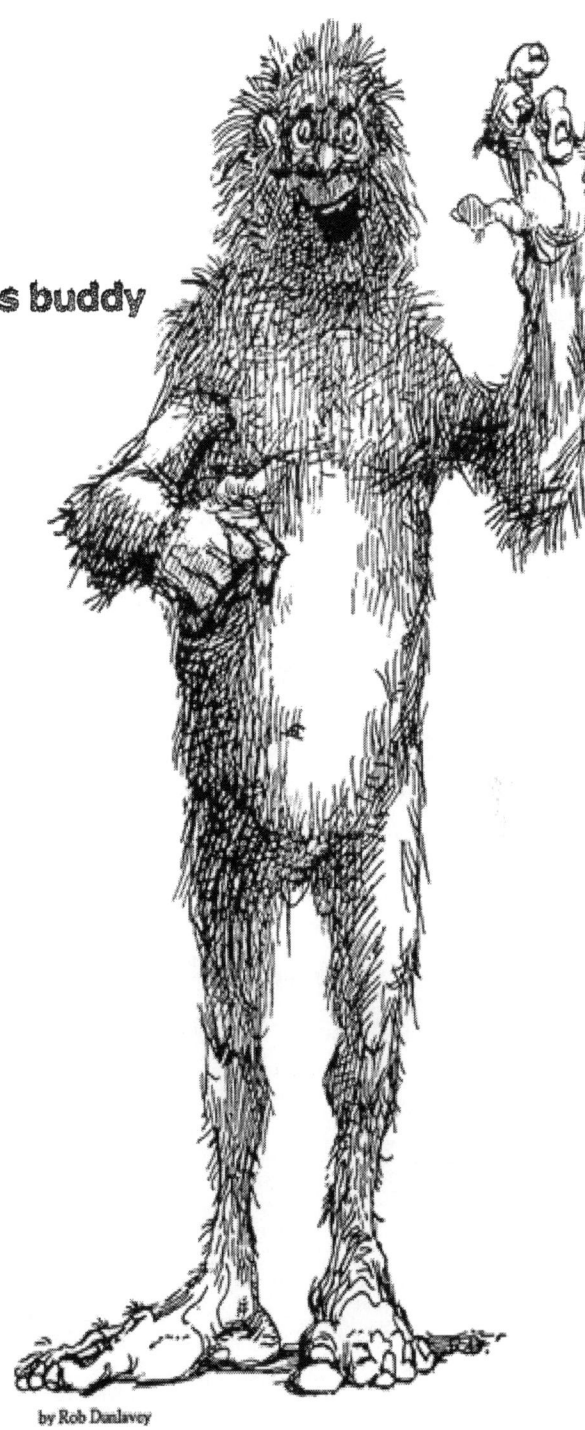

ROGAINING EXCUSE T-SHIRT

I THOUGHT IT WAS A HAIR TONIC

TOO MANY CONTOURS IN FIRST 60K

FOLLOWED ANOTHER TEAM OFF THE MAP

DRINKING WATER TOO HOT

BLISTERS OVERCAME AMBITIOUS PLAN

COMPASS POINTED TO KNIFE, MOSTLY

180-DEGREE ERROR

AIMED OFF–TOO FAR OFF

PARTNER BLUNDERED–CHOSE ME

THEY RAN OUT OF CHILI!

HEADLAMP FAILED–LAST ROGAINE'S BATTERIES

YELLOW JACKETS OBJECTED TO MY ROUTE

BEAR CUBS ON MY TRAIL–BUT MOTHER?

WHISTLE FULL OF DIRT FROM FALL

DRY CROSSING WASN'T

UNCROSSABLE SWAMP WAS

FULL MOON LASTED 15 MINUTES

MY TENT BLEW INTO LAKE

MISSED CONTROL LATER SPOTTED FROM A MILE AWAY

MY INDESTRUCTIBLE BOOTS WEREN'T

PARTNER FOUND NEW WAY TO GET LOST

SAND IN SANDWICH

DSQ–SPLIT FOR PIT STOP

SLEPT THROUGH PLANNED NIGHT LOOP

UNCROSSABLE CLIFF WAS

LOST SHOE IN GOPHER HOLE

THEY TOLD ME ROGAINE MEANT FLAT TERRAIN

WATER FILTER PLUGGED WITH TADPOLES

HOT CHILI HAD PREDICTABLE RESULTS

ATTACKED BY KILLER GRASS SEEDS

FOLLOWED FROG CROAKS TO WRONG SWAMP

BULL PATROLLING CONTROL IN PASTURE

PARTNER DOWN WITH DIAPER RASH

THE CLEARINGS WEREN'T

SUN COOKED PARTNER'S BRAINS

WAIT-A-MINUTE BUSHES EVERYWHERE

FIRST 50 KM AT 4 KPH, LAST 40 AT ZERO

PARALLELED UNMAPPED TRAIL FOR 2 KM

LAUREL HELLS WERE JUST THAT

14 OF 24 HOURS AT HASH HOUSE

THOUGHT WE SAW A SASQUATCH

This T-Shirt was used for the Tamarack Spring Rogaine, United States Rogaining Championships, September 14-15, 2002.

ORDER OF THE GEODUCK

Order of the Geoduck is an international award issued by the International Rogaining Federation for long-term high-level contributions to international rogaining.

Geoduck Awardees:

1994 Carl Moore (United States)
1995 Keg Good (United States)
1996 Eric Smith (United States)
1997 Wilkey Richardson (United States)
1998 Murray Foubister (Canada)
1999 Michael Haynes (Canada)
2000 Michael Wood (New Zealand)
2001 Peg Davis (United States)
2002 Neil Phillips (Australia)
2003 Rod Phillips (Australia)
2004 John Maier (United States)
2005 Andres Käär (Estonia)
2006 Mal Harding (United States)
2006 Alan Mansfield (Australia)
2006 Mike Sheridan (New Zealand)
2007 Francis Falardeau (Canada)
2008 Peter Taylor (Australia)
2008 Peter Squires (New Zealand)
2010 Bill Kennedy (New Zealand)
2010: Derek Morris (Australia).
2012 Lauri Leppik (Estonia)
2012 Bob Reddick (United States)
2014 Efim Shtempler (Ukraine)
2016 Sergey Yashchenko (Russia)
2020 Jan Tojnar (Czech Republic)
2020 Richard Robinson (Australia)

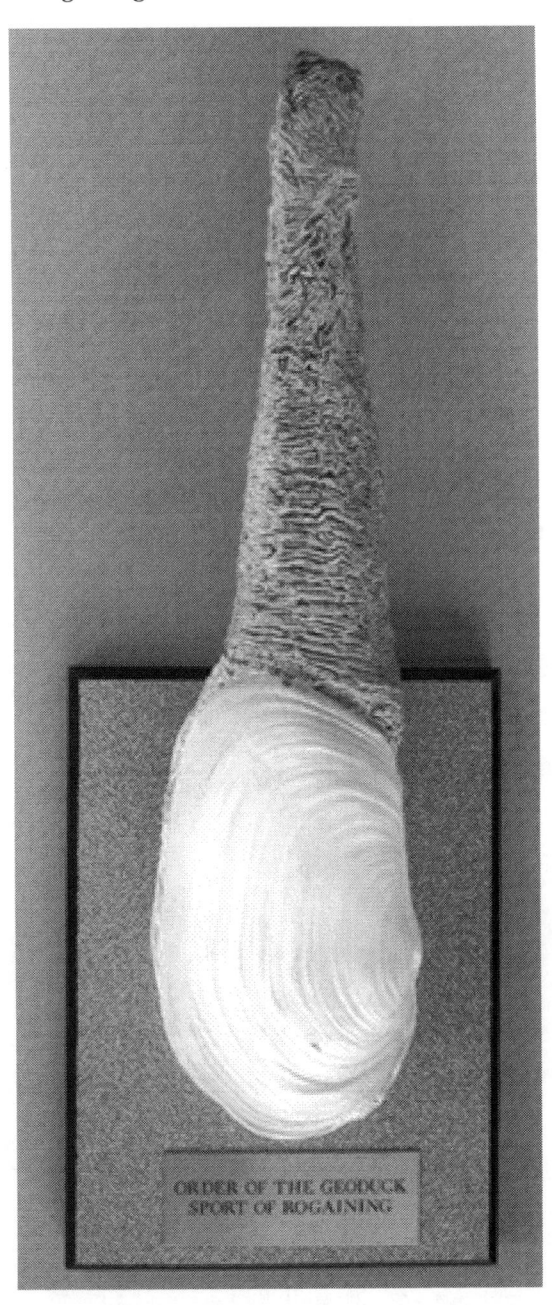

BLACK HILLS WRC SEARCH AND RESCUE—FOR REAL

Two weeks prior to the WRC14, meet director Rick Emerson worked on a test search and rescue scenario which said that a team at night had a person with a broken ankle, and that another rogainer with a cell phone had gone some distance to a hilltop to call in the emergency, with all location references to control bag sites. Eerily, almost the identical thing happened for real, and to my team!

The safety, medical, and search and rescue people, Gwen, Jessica, Jeremy, Vicki, and Tracy Fraterelli worked in the medical tent and went out on road patrols on 2-hour shifts. A few teams were helped: lots of scrapes from downed trees, a head laceration, and a swollen (possibly fractured) forearm. The cuts were treated in the field and a make-shift splint/wrap placed on the arm and away everyone went. Rogainers tend be gnarly types, not eager to quit.

The first medical tent visitor slowly walked/puked in around 8 PM. He was lightheaded, shivering, vomiting, and exhausted. Couldn't keep a thing down. Small cut on a finger. After 2 hours of rest, ice chips, and bites of banana he felt better, but was out of the race. His two other teammates were still out on the course having fun. Two others came in with the same symptoms: vomiting, cramping, lightheaded, shivering, and exhaustion. They just needed to rest and slowly replenish fluids. Not much further action until 4 AM, when a cell phone call (mine) at last got through to Tracy.

The senior (combined ages 240) Mixed Ultravet Sasqwatchers team of Ken Lew, Pat Reddick, and I tried to do one more control #70 before nightfall Saturday. Our plan was to return to the Hash House (aka start/finish) for dinner about 8 PM, sleep on cots there instead of our usual return to our B&B, and do more controls after breakfast.

We had light jackets, hats, and trail food, but were not fully prepared for an overnight bivouac. Our efforts to find #70 failed and we did not find the control in the steep reentrant, with lots of downed timber, as night fell. I was surprised then to suddenly lose most all of my balance after dark, even using a good LED headlamp and a flashlight. I needed that visual input, since my old numb feet (peripheral neuropathy) condition was disabling. Ken was doing well, so I followed him. Pat had worn stylish slip-on footwear which worked for her, until it didn't.

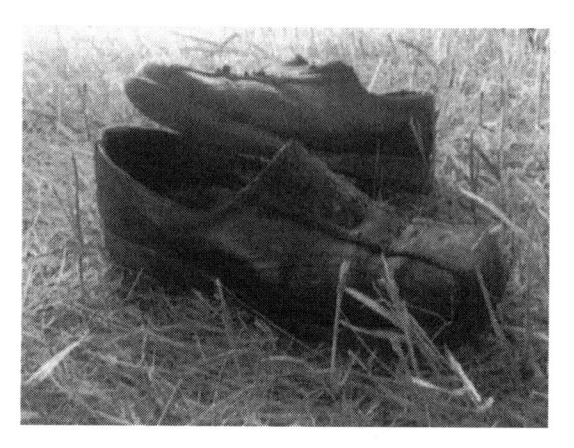

We gave up on #70 and tried to bail out to do a 5 kilometer moonlight walk on a level horse trail back to the hash house. I had forgotten to zip on the pant legs to my hiking shorts, so collected lots of scratches on both legs. Ken and I were each using two hiking poles. We were heading west, downhill, and on the safety bearing certain to hit the horse trail and highway very soon, bailing out to the end. We soon turned south to avoid any uphill, and it looked like a long but easy walk in the moonlight!

So there we went, trekking downhill into hidden, muddy, boggy terrain, Ken leading, me staggering, and Pat losing her shoes twice in deep mud. Besides a very snowy winter in the Black Hills, there had recently been five inches of rain, turning the reentrant we were following downward into a hidden grass-covered swamp of mud.

We soon reversed to an uphill track to firmer ground and were somewhere ½ way between #20 and #70 in thick woods and deadfall. Ken scouted ahead as I found it safer to crawl, and then we were about to go for a dry path exit, when Ken tripped over roots and deadfall on a downhill slope and fell backwards right in front of me. He struck his head with a resounding bang on a tree, and landed with his head trapped between it and a log.

Pat and I got him free with difficulty by lifting the log, and then we asked that he lie down and be still until we could see his condition. We all then voted to open my sealed cell phone (a DSQ-ing act) and call for extraction at about 1:30 AM. It took minutes to cut open the double-sealed packet with a small scissors and pen knife. My first of some 28 calls went nowhere in a very weak cell phone signal area, so I crawled to a higher elevation, found a 1-bar and sometimes a 2-bar signal, and after many message machines and call drops, I reached Rick at about 2:34 AM, then Tracy. I stayed up there to make more calls.

After my first contact, Tracy launched volunteers Sean, Scott, and Gary who, backed up by the Lawrence County Search and Rescue team, responded with searches initially to a poor GPS reading I had obtained, which was in error by some 4/5th of a mile.

I used an app called Flashlight on my cell phone to flash around the tree tops above me. Searchers were blowing whistles, likely south of #70, but nothing was heard by us. Later, we found out the searchers just then saw flashing lights over near #105, which was about 2 km. east of us. That drew them off from very near us.

It was coldest, perhaps 49 degrees, at 6100 feet elevation just at dawn, and we were all shivering by that time. The only whistle I heard all night was Pat's, at about 4:30 AM. We were separated by perhaps only 50 meters, but I could barely hear her whistle through the woods. We were not where a passing rogaining team might find us.

Pat got a little sleep at first while waiting, but also was concerned about the lightning visible on the horizon, and the reports of a mountain lion. A female team had approached a control and saw two reflectors shining, but one of them was the eye of a mountain lion sitting under the control. It later followed a team for a while. The park ranger had announced that some 200 mountain lions were residents of the park.

Pat kept an eye on Ken who was constantly shivering and groaning. We had wrapped him in a bivy sack as best we could, and put two inflatable pillows under him. She also worried about me not coming back after trying to make calls.

A better GPS reading and further cell calls got the searchers redirected back NW of #70, and then my battery went dead. Gary, Scott, Sean, and Steve found us at 6:45 AM.

They were not initially carrying in water (I got a ½ pint of cold hot cocoa and scarfed down some crackers, and later some water from a searchers water bladder and Gary's warm sweater). Ken got some crackers and more blankets.

With daylight, I could balance enough to walk again, and Pat and I were separately walked out by volunteers to vehicles for trips back to the Hash House and breakfast. Ken, however, was shivering, complaining of pains and suspected by Leslie to have a broken hip, so EMS was called at 7:10 AM. Leslie, Mark, Sean, and the SAR folks took over from there, using chain saws to cut a path down the hill to take Ken out. Ken was carried out on a board by four men to a trailer, then to a helicopter, and then off to the Rapid City Regional Hospital. As they bundled him up on the hillside, he asked, "Can someone take my picture first?"

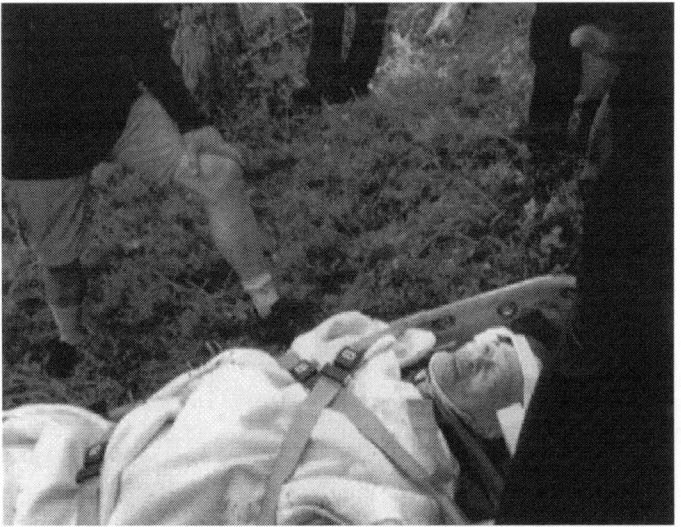

Ken got a smooth, speedy ride, but saw only sky during the flight. Pat was fine, but I got checked carefully for blood pressure (very high) and wounds at the medical tent. I got a tiny bandage on my right fourth toe and no sympathy at all for my scraped up lower legs. Tracy washed Pat's limbs with poison ivy treatment soap, in case of exposure. She was surprised that all three of us seemed to take this incident without complaint and in stride, as if it was a regular part of rogaining.

While waiting for the award ceremony, I bought a clean event map which became a giant get-well card for Ken, with signatures and notes added from many teams.

Pat and I saw Ken at his hospital room Monday afternoon, just as the hip surgeon first came in to tell him that the CAT scan disputed the X-ray that had maybe shown a hairline fracture, and that the good news was that there was no break. Good-looking nurses were hovering around, giving Ken lots of TLC. He did have a sore tailbone, a sore spot on his head, but no skull or brain injury, and a sore leg due to a 5-lb. weight tractioning his foot in case of a hip break.

To our surprise, Ken was released Tuesday evening without further treatment. So, we all went shopping the next morning in Rapid City and flew back as scheduled Wednesday. Ken treasured his get-well card and hand-carried it carefully on the flights back home to Seattle.

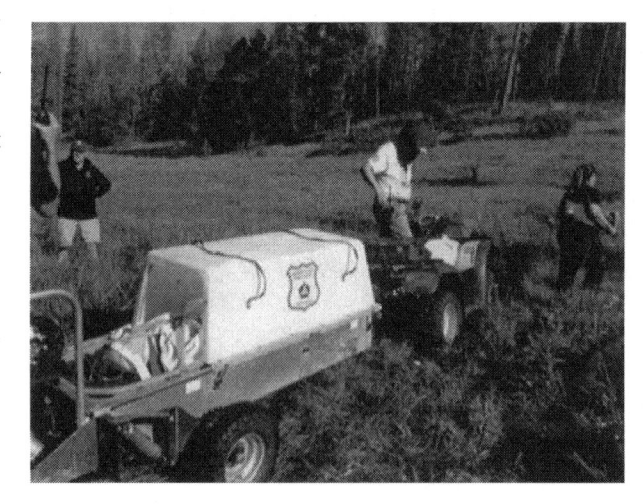

Ken is now walking better than I am, in good humor, and has been seen by his own doctor, who told him to take it easy around the house and not to drive for a while. Meanwhile, my doctor has found a retinal vein blockage in my right eye (unrelated to rogaining?), and I've had a shot in the eyeball to medicate it. Pat with great patience tolerates all this male inadequacy around here, but is taking long naps to try to match mine. Her shoes are now archived in the photo history of the WRC.

Our team voted unanimously to retire the notorious Sasqwatchers from active rogaining competition, after 7 WRCs in six countries, and change to a spectator role, which has had very few people in attendance at WRCs. Our thanks go to all the rescue teams, the helicopter crew, and the rogaine support staff who performed outstandingly.

(Tracy Fraterelli and Sean Fehey contributed to this report.)

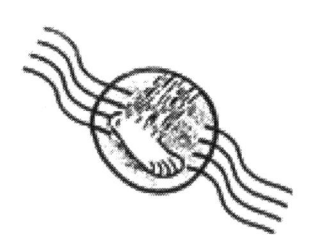

Answers to Youngsters in the Back Yard quiz on page 98: 5, 4, 3, 2

Made in the USA
Columbia, SC
21 May 2023